Have you been fooled by t of healthcare violence

Myth #1: If you say something, it will make things worse

Myth #2: Don't sweat the small stuff

Myth #3: Kill them with kindness

Myth #4: People behave badly because they are sick and under stress

Myth #5: Violence is just part of the job

Myth #6: The customer is always right

Myth #7: Things really aren't that bad

If you think any of these are true, how you behave as a result is likely compromising your safety and the safety of others.

In this book, Joel Lashley, a recognized authority on healthcare violence, invalidates these myths and explains how to create environments of care that are incompatible with anti-social and aggressive behavior.

Confidence In Conflict For Healthcare Professionals not only offers strategies hospitals and clinics can implement system-wide, but also describes concrete steps individual caregivers can take immediately to create safer and more therapeutic provider/patient relationships.

The book explores the range of healthcare violence – from disrespect, to intimidation, to physical assaults – and the effect violence has on caregiver injuries, employee morale, patient satisfaction, clinical outcomes and the financial bottom line of healthcare institutions. It then guides the reader through the process of creating environments of care that are incompatible with violence.

It's no longer acceptable to allow the epidemic of healthcare violence to continue.

Confidence
IN / CONFLICT
FOR HEALTHCARE PROFESSIONALS
Creating an Environment Of Care That Is Incompatible With Violence

By: Joel Lashley

With: Mike Thiel and Bob Willis

Truths Publishing
Milwaukee, WI

Dedication

This book is dedicated to my wife, Amanda, the best crisis communicator I ever met.

To my son Colin, who taught me my most important lessons about how to communicate under pressure.

To my mother Anna, who has spent a lifetime helping those in need.

And finally to my father, Norman, who often said I should write a book. Okay Dad, here it is.

www.ConfidenceInConflict.com

For bulk-purchasing pricing, please contact:
  Vistelar
  1845 N. Farwell Ave., Suite 210
  Milwaukee, WI 53202
  Phone: 877-690-8230
  Fax: 866-406-2374
  Email: info@vistelar.com
  Web: www.vistelar.com

Joel Lashley
Confidence In Conflict For Healthcare Professionals / Joel Lashley
Contributors:
  • Robert C. (Bob) Willis, Consultant
  • Mike Thiel, Director of Security, Children's Hospital of Wisconsin

Edited by Allen Oelschlaeger
Revised Edition 2017

ISBN 13: 978-0-9909109-1-6
ISBN 10: 0-9909109-1-1
LCCN: 2015953697

BISAC Subject Headings:
  MEDICAL / Nursing / Management & Leadership
  MEDICAL / Health Care Delivery
  MEDICAL / Nursing / Issues
  MEDICAL / Education & Training

Published By Truths Publishing, Milwaukee, WI
Printed In the United States of America

Table of Contents

Joel Lashley

Foreword
by Mike Thiel

We all know what acts of violence look like; shootings, stabbings, assaults, injuries, arrests, victims, death, body counts. And, in the aftermath of violence, there's much more that plays out over time; medical care, survival stories, shooter histories, fear, blame. It's a sequence we know all too well, like some horrific movie that we've watched over and over so many times we can recite the lines by heart. We know what happens next and yet we anxiously watch to see how it ends; justice, healing, forgiving and never forgetting.

But violence doesn't just happen. When we review the entire sequence of events leading up to the last acts, we readily recognize a series of behaviors and events that lead down the path and set the stage for violence—those behaviors that offer clues into what was coming; conflict, broken relationships, antisocial behaviors, implied threats, social media postings, explicit threats. We try to explain the spiral into violence as a simple cause and effect relationship. If someone had done something differently at a specific point in the timeline, the violent outcome would have never materialized. Hindsight is always 20/20. It's easy to recognize the first acts of violence when we know how the movie ends.

1

In *Confidence In Conflict for Healthcare Professionals*, you will learn how to change the movie script. That said, human beings are complicated and we don't often follow a script. What triggers one person to lash out may not have the same effect on others. Behaviors tolerated by one social group may be abhorrent and disrespectful to another. However, the ultimate response to conflict and violence within an institution is determined by its own unique culture or social contract. A culture incompatible with violence is a culture where violence can't take hold, because conflict is best resolved in the incipient stage. How to create such an institutional culture is what you'll learn in *Confidence In Conflict For Healthcare Professionals*.

As the Director of Security at a level one trauma center, I know that violence comes to healthcare. Whether it's medical care, psychiatric care, outpatient treatment or social services, violence in the community usually ends up at the doorstep of a hospital. While the media draws attention to homicide, the vast majority of violence in the workplace results in non-fatal, yet serious injury. And more of it happens to healthcare providers than anyone else.

Building a healthcare culture incompatible with violence is not easy. It feels overwhelming. But we have to start somewhere. This book explores the environment of healthcare and shares what works and what doesn't. At its core, what works is infusing dignity by showing respect into every single interaction in healthcare to create an environment incompatible with violence. We know that's not the culture in healthcare today, so something must change—and this book shows us how.

Communicating under pressure is a learned process and we certainly know communication tactics can be learned. We all learn how to argue at an early age. Any two-year old can easily convince you they have mastered the art of debate. How quickly we learn to use words to lie, disguise our feelings, or simply raise our voice to intimidate the competition. We learn how to use curse words, we learn how to threaten and we learn how to defend ourselves. But, that's not the learning we need. Instead we need to learn how to communicate in a way that treats others with dignity by showing them respect. That's what you will learn in this book.

Joel Lashley

Introduction
The Big, Mean, Angry Biker
Communicating Under Pressure

"Human nature is complex. Even if we have inclinations toward violence,
we also have inclination to empathy, to cooperation, to self-control."
Steven Pinker

I was passing through the Emergency Department when an angry looking man walked in through the front door. He was a hard figure to miss. He wore a denim jacket with the sleeves torn off and emblazoned on his makeshift vest were the colors of a well-known and notoriously violent motorcycle gang. His bare arms were heavily inked with gang colors, lewd images, swastikas, and various weapons.

He was at least six and a half feet tall and easily weighed over 300 pounds. His long bushy hair flowed over his shoulders. His beard was equally impressive, reaching all the way down to his pistol-shaped belt buckle. His wide black belt was encrusted with pointed metal studs and a long heavy chrome chain secured his wallet to it. His jeans were tucked into his tall studded motorcycle boots, which could easily have concealed a knife or small-framed handgun.

The big man stood in the lobby with his feet apart, his huge fists clenched, and wearing an obvious look of disgust on his face. Without saying a word, he commanded the room as all eyes were on him. Finally he shouted, "Where am I supposed to park my f***ing van?!" You could have heard a pin drop. Everyone in the room froze, staff and patients alike.

I was dressed in a suit and didn't look particularly intimidating. Still, I decided to address the big man. I walked towards him with a look of confident concern on my face, because when people are angry they don't want to be smiled at. I didn't stand directly in front of him. Instead, I stood about ten feet away with my feet apart and my hands out in front of me. At ten feet, I could quickly *evaluate* or *exit* the scene if he suddenly flew off the handle. As soon as I was in position, I began to speak.

"Hello, Sir. I'm Joel. I work here in the hospital." Now the big man looked directly at me. "I can help you with your van, but can I ask you not to yell or curse? There are kids and families around. Let me help you out." The man looked at me with an expression of angry shock. In my peripheral vision, I could see nurses backing away and seeking safety. After a short pause, he spoke again. This time more quietly.

"Whatever." he replied. "Where am I supposed to park around here? The lot is full." Based on his initial reaction to me, I closed some of the space between us to about five feet so we could communicate more effectively without crowding each other. At five feet, I could more effectively *communicate or evade* an attack should things go badly.

"You're in luck." I answered. "Let me get a valet to park your car. Valet service is free here."

"I don't want anyone driving my f***ing van!" he shouted back. "I don't need anyone else in my f***ing van!" Clearly he wasn't getting the message, so I continued.

"Sir, I have to ask you again not to yell or curse. There are patients and children around and this has to be a safe place for them. You're a big guy and you're scaring everybody. We can't allow that in the hospital, so please stop."

The big biker looked down at me and sighed, before answering me in a strained whisper. "Whatever. Where can I park, then?" Now satisfied that he was going to cooperate, I moved up within two feet of him so we could talk without compromising patient confidentiality. Two feet is the distance at where I could *operate or escape*, if necessary. First, I asked him if he was in need of emergency care. He explained that he was here to visit his son. I asked him his son's name and checked with the triage nurse to make certain the child was in the Emergency Department and that there was no dire medical emergency. The biker became visibly calmer, because *information equals peace*. One of the main reasons people act-out in clinical situations is fear or frustration linked to a misunderstanding or a lack of basic information.

Then came the hard part. I told him that, if he didn't want to use the valet service, he would have to park several blocks away on the other side of the campus. He would then have to come through the main hospital entrance. Once there, he would have to get a visitor pass and directions back to the emergency department. Of course, that made him angry again. "Whatever. This is ridiculous," he snarled under his breath, but this time without cursing or yelling. He then turned and walked back out into the parking lot.

Several minutes later the big, mean, angry biker appeared at the visitors' center in the main lobby. There were a lot of people in line, so he soon lost his temper. "This is ridiculous," he yelled! "How do I get to the f***ing emergency room from here? I don't have time for this bulls***!" The security officer assigned to the hospital lobby overheard him and didn't waste any time responding. Being mindful of his *proxemics*, i.e., managing his distance to the subject depending on the level of threat, he approached with caution and began *evaluating* the subject at ten feet away. When he was satisfied that the big biker was unarmed and not actively aggressive, he approached with caution up to five feet where he could *communicate*. Then he stood and spoke as trained.

"Sir, I'm Mark, with security".

"So?" replied the biker, rolling his eyes.

"I will help you get to the emergency department, but please stop cursing and yelling. We have to keep things quiet and peaceful in the hospital for the patients."

The big biker snarled back, saying "Are you for real?"

Now relaxed but ready at five feet away, the officer simply smiled and continued, "Look, you're going to give some heart patient another heart attack! We have to keep things calm around here."

To that, the big biker finally smirked and shook his head. Then he replied, using his word of choice. "Whatever. Just get me over there, will you?" The officer then stayed on track, now *operating* at two feet he made sure everything was in order before taking the biker to the Emergency Department.

"My pleasure. First we have to get you a pass. Who are you here to see today?" While the security officer assisted the big biker, I was waiting back at the Emergency Department to see what would happen when the big biker showed up again. When he finally arrived, it was the triage nurses' turn with him.

"Hello, I'm Amy. I'm the nurse who is checking in your son. I have to ask you some questions about him. It should only take a few minutes. First, how do you spell his first name?"

The big biker looked annoyed again, "Are you kidding? His name is Jerry."

"Jerry or Gerald" she continued, unshaken.

The biker looked puzzled, "Uh, Gerald"

"With a G or a J?" she asked.

"J, I think." answered the biker, "Isn't that in his records or something?"

"Oh sure," said the nurse. "That is if he's been here before. We need proper spelling to find his record or it will take much longer. Now, how do you spell his last name?" To that, the biker obediently spelled out the boy's last name. Then she continued to question the biker, "Is he on any medications?"

"Isn't that in the records, either?" he asked.

"Possibly, but your boy may have been prescribed new meds by his doctor, since he was last here. We need that information to keep him safe."

The big biker answered, but continued to do what uncooperative people do. He challenged every question and resisted every step. In response, the nurse did what trained and capable communicators do when they meet verbal resistance: used *Redirections*. She was clearly a master of this tactic. She *deflected* all his resistance by acknowledging each question, while still keeping the biker on track. And she did it with one simple word, the word "*but.*"

When she was finished, she sent the biker over to registration. He refused to sit when the young registration woman offered him a seat, so she just started in with her questions. "How do you spell your child's name?" The biker grew visibly annoyed again.

"Are you kidding? Can't you just ask her?" while gesturing toward the triage nurse.

"Yes, but she's with another patient right now. Can I just ask you for his name again, please? Then I can quickly verify his address and insurance." The young woman did a very nice job of using the *Redirections* tactic and keeping the biker on track, just as the nurse had done. All seemed to be going along smoothly, until the young woman advised him that he wasn't the father of record. Finally, he began to shout again.

"That's not right! I pay this kid's bills!" Because the biker was shouting again, his behavior had to be readdressed. That said, there was still a noticeable change in the biker's behavior. He wasn't cursing. Even after this stumble, he was still actively modifying his normal behavior.

When he began to shout, the young woman rolled back in her chair a few feet and kept the counter between them, as trained. She then replied by simply stating, "Sir, please don't shout. There are sick people and kids around, and you're making them feel unsafe." Her expression was concerned and her tone of voice was professional and confident. The biker stopped yelling, but continued in a low volume.

"That ain't right!" he whispered hoarsely. The registration person also explained that, since he wasn't a legal guardian or adoptive parent, he could not give permission to treat. The biker was now beside himself with anger. "I'm going to sue this place," he whispered angrily. "I can't believe this!" His face was red and he pointed his finger at the registration person, as he raged on in whispered tones.

The registration person kept the counter between them and stayed out of reach, while he quietly vented. She *empathized* by saying, "I understand that you're angry, but our hands are tied because it's the law. Help me get a hold of his mother, so we can make sure he gets all the care he needs as quickly as possible. In the meantime, they will care for him as necessary, until we can get a hold of her."

With that, the biker calmed down enough to answer the rest of her questions. She then gestured towards the waiting area and asked him to take a seat. But, if you know anything about tough guys, no one tells them to sit down, especially women! So he stood there like a statue, unmoving and waiting for someone to take him back in the treatment area to see his girlfriend's son.

After a few tense seconds, the registration person simply looked up at the man and confidently stated, "Sir, can I ask you again to take a seat, please? I assure you that they will call you soon. I have other people waiting in line." At that, the biker looked around the room at all the faces he hadn't taken notice of before. Some of them were staring uncomfortably off into space. Others looked at him with a puzzled or disgusted expression. Then he simply turned, walked to the waiting area, and sat down.

With things settled down for the time being, I went back to the treatment area to advise the medical staff about what had just transpired. They assured me that they would call security quickly if the man started up again, as his behavior had already been addressed several times. I then went on to my meeting.

A couple of hours later, I walked back to the emergency department to see how things were going. I asked the doctor how the big biker was doing. "He's fine. No problems. You shouldn't judge a book by its cover, you know," he said smugly. I then went to the nurse who was working with the boy, his mother and the biker. She described the big biker as "pleasant." When the biker left later that day, he stopped by the visitors' center and apologized to the people working there, stating that he was sorry he'd behaved like a jerk. Then the formerly big, mean, angry biker, his girlfriend, and her son walked out towards the parking lot.

What could account for such a transformation? Was it his girlfriend perhaps? Not likely, she hadn't shown up until way after the biker had been given permission to see the boy. The nurse also said he'd already become "pleasant" long before his girlfriend arrived. So then what could account for the change? Perhaps we can figure it out by asking what he may have been like, if he'd been handled a different way.

Would the biker's behavior have changed, if I'd ignored him and allowed him to yell and curse? Would it have gotten worse or better? Perhaps I could have told him just to leave his car parked in a no parking zone and not to worry about it. That might have appeased him, until he got a parking ticket. Appeasement rarely works anyway. Mike Thiel, the Director of Security at Children's Hospital of Wisconsin likes to put it this way: "appeasement equals encouragement for more bad behavior." Also, mere appeasement doesn't address the underlying problem.

When we fail to resolve problems, in favor of ignoring them, they usually become bigger problems. Still, this is the direction we usually go when we encounter anti-social and even threatening behavior in hospitals and clinics. We follow the path of least resistance to get the angry and threatening person out of our way; and following the path of least resistance almost always leads to failure.

What if when he questioned the triage procedure, the nurse offered to simply wait and ask the child's mother when she arrived? Might that have worked? Or would she have placed the patient in greater danger, by not having timely information about medications, food intake, conditions, allergies, and etcetera? Also, that would be just more appeasement, i.e., more validation of the illusion that bad behavior gets results.

If the registration person had just let the biker vent, as she'd heard people say before, would he have gotten everything off his chest and been fine, or would his bad behavior have escalated? If at every step, the biker had been treated with kid gloves, given a wide berth, and killed with kindness—in other words, embraced all the advice nurses are given throughout their careers—would he have turned into this nice pleasant man they encountered in the treatment area or would he have been something entirely different?

In reality, he would have been taken down a path towards violence. He would have continued to be loud, obnoxious, and threatening. As a result, other patients and families would have been disturbed, the emergency medical staff would have become fearful, and the patient would have been over-stimulated. When other patients and families are disturbed, they complain and even consider going elsewhere for their medical care. When medical staff becomes fearful, they experience more stress and many consider seeking new employment. Worst of all, medical staff may spend less time with patients and make more mistakes. The hospital loses, the staff loses, and patients lose.

Appeasement in the face of anti-social and threatening behavior is the path we most often take in human service work, all because of a mythology that exists about violence in our workplace and how it should be handled. That is, a mythology that directs us to legitimize and even reward anti-social and threatening behavior. What are these myths? Why do we continue to embrace them and pass them on, even in the face of so many failures? First we need to recognize what these myths are, before we can go in another direction.

Also, we have to ask ourselves, does the biker behave this way in all situations and in all places? Would he have behaved the same way in a church or a library? Perhaps, but it's not a foregone conclusion. Can we assume that, if he behaved that way in a library or church, he wouldn't be welcome there?

So what made the intervention with the angry biker successful? What stands out most is the consistent response from the staff. *Inconsistency is the enemy of peace.* Consistency, on the other hand, is the basis for all successful intervention and the ultimate exclusion of unwanted behavior within a relationship or group.

The "Big, Mean, Angry Biker" story is just one of thousands from my thirty-plus years of work in public safety. I've repeatedly encountered people just like him and I've seen the good the bad and the ugly that can result from the wide range of approaches used to address challenging behaviors like his.

I first got into the security field in 1981 and began my career in healthcare security in 1985 at a large urban residential and sub-acute care facility. Since then, I've worked in everything from small community based social service agencies to busy urban medical centers.

For 18 years, I worked at Children's Hospital of Wisconsin, where I finished out my service as the security training coordinator for the security, healthcare, social services and behavioral health staff and other providers from virtually all disciplines. During my tenure there, I had the privilege to learn from many wonderful mentors, including Mike Thiel (who wrote the Foreword to this book), Dr. George Thompson (founder of the Verbal Judo Institute), Gary Klugiewicz (co-founder of Vistelar) and countless nurses, doctors, behavioral health therapists, all types of other healthcare professionals, patients and their parents. Together, we transformed the environment of care for everyone — provider and patient alike.

Currently, I work at Aurora Health Care where I supervise security operations for community clinics in Wisconsin. Aurora is a large integrated healthcare provider with over 31,000 employees, 15 hospitals, over 150 clinic sites and more than 7.5 million annual patient encounters.

In addition, I am a Law Enforcement Crisis Intervention Teams Instructor for the National Alliance on Mental Illness (NAMI), and a member of the International Law Enforcement Educators and Trainers Association (ILEETA).

In 2005 I was introduced to the Vistelar's conflict management methodologies, which you'll learn about in this book. The class I attended was co-taught by Gary Klugiewicz, a professional trainer who began teaching verbal intervention skills to police officers in the early 1980s.

Gary and some others formed a company called Vistelar in 2009 to bring these verbal intervention principles and other conflict management training to other disciplines beyond law enforcement, including healthcare. Shortly thereafter, I became a Certified Consultant for Vistelar, which I still am today.

Vistelar is a consulting and training institute focused on addressing the entire spectrum of human conflict at the point of impact—from before an interaction begins through to the consequences of how an interaction is managed. A lot of what you'll learn in this book is embedded in Vistelar's conflict management training curriculum.

Several years ago I began telling the "Big, Mean, Angry Biker" story to everyone who would listen. I told it at every nursing orientation for every newly hired RN and nursing assistant. I told it at every nursing in-service I taught. I shared the story to providers in the emergency department, critical care units, urgent care clinics, doctor's offices, day surgery clinics, renal clinics, social service agencies, and psychiatric clinics. Anywhere and everywhere that people were concerned with reducing disruptive behavior and violence within their walls, I shared this story.

Soon, I ended up taking this story and the concepts it represents, such as *Gateway Behaviors of Violence, Social Contracting* and *Crisis Intervention* on the road, as calls came in from national healthcare and campus safety organizations. I've taught these principles all over the country, not only in hospitals but also at police departments, schools, and even jails.

Everywhere the "Big Mean, Angry, Biker" story and I went, I saw it transform the minds of people who are steeped in violence daily and at a total loss for what to do about it. I don't know the biker's name, but if I did, I'd like to shake his hand and thank him for teaching me some of the most important lessons I ever learned. I like to think he learned something from that experience as well.

Everyone who works in healthcare needs to know this story and learn what we did to turn the biker on a different path — a path towards peace for providers and patients, and a better patient experience for himself. My primary goal with this book is to share the lessons I've learned over the last three decades with individual healthcare providers who, every day, face disrespect and violence.

Disrespect and violence — they no longer have to be accepted as just "part of the job."

Chapter One
How Much Danger Am I In?
Be Alert and Decisive

"Only human beings can look directly at something, have all the information they need to make an accurate prediction, perhaps even momentarily make the accurate prediction, and then say that it isn't so."

Gavin de Becker

Though it rarely occurs to anyone entering the healthcare field that they might experience high levels of conflict and violence, soon after beginning their clinical training providers are taught to accept a culture of violence. That's because the culture of healthcare embraces the belief that violence is part of the job. From one certainly tragic point of view the people who embrace this notion are absolutely right. Violence is a day-to-day reality in healthcare.

How bad is the problem? Among the ranks of risk management professionals workplace violence is a much talked about issue. But is workplace violence an even larger issue in healthcare? If the federal government's own statistics from sources such as the Bureau of Labor Statistics are to be believed, *healthcare is the most violent profession in the private sector.* According the bureau 45% of all nonfatal assaults against workers resulting in time away from work occur in the healthcare industry.

OSHA estimates that there are approximately 2,600 non-fatal assaults on hospital staff annually. This estimate does not include homicides. Nurses, nursing assistants and hospital security officers are victimized the most, but no one in a hospital is immune. Everyone from physicians to pharmacists is assaulted on the job at higher than average rates. As one might expect, emergency medicine, critical care, and psychiatry top the list, but violence can and does happen anywhere in a hospital or clinic. In fact, hospital admissions and registration staff are also at elevated risk.

The levels of violence in healthcare is not going unnoticed by the CDC, OSHA, the Joint Commission and other agencies concerned with the health and well being of healthcare workers. In 2010, a Joint Commission Alert advised that healthcare workers need to take increased measures to curb the levels of violence in hospitals. Most significant perhaps is the alerts' acknowledgement that violent crime is increasing in the healthcare setting and that workers, patients, and visitors are all at increased risk.

One of the more prevalent misperceptions is that these grim statistics, particularly those sourced from the Bureau of Labor Statistics, include numbers of minor assaults, such as shoves or spitting incidents. Nothing could be further from the truth. In order to qualify for the government's statistics, workers must have suffered enough of an injury to miss time from work. We can place these numbers into an even clearer perspective by accepting the following reality. None of these statistics represent all of the so called "minor" assaults, such as slaps, shoves, unwanted sexual touching, spitting, verbal threats, and other assaults that do not result in time off from work. This represents an even greater number of uncounted assaults, because healthcare workers are notorious for accepting and underreporting violent incidents. Police officers and prison guards are not so forgiving and rightly so.

In their groundbreaking surveys between 2009 and 2012, the Emergency Nurses Association discovered that half of all emergency department nurses surveyed have been the target of violence and threats on the job. Also, half of those who reported said they had experienced twenty or more violent and/or threatening incidents during their last three years on the job. Overall, even according to the government's statistics, which are limited to assaults resulting in injury, around *20,000 registered nurses are assaulted annually and over 40,000 nursing assistants!* Physicians, respiratory therapists, hospital security officers, x-ray technicians, social workers, and many others are also assaulted at unusually high rates.

The loss of quality healthcare workers due to violence related turnover and the hundreds of millions of dollars lost annually from injuries are devastating. In a very real way violence in healthcare has become one of the medical profession's biggest problems and can no longer be contained as one of its dirty little secrets.

The following story is a blatant example — albeit an all too familiar one — of a level of acceptance that is perhaps unique to healthcare. While merely engaged in a casual conversation, a law enforcement professional asked a healthcare professional how her day was going. She related that moments earlier she had almost been sexually assaulted. This nurse practitioner was able to escape from the situation by having done an appropriate assessment and using some evasive tactics.

After escaping the potentially catastrophic attack, she told the shocked police officer that the police were not contacted and that she simply went to a location where others were present and waited for her attacker to leave the scene. She did say that she notified her supervisor and documented the incident in the patient's medical record. The scariest part of the whole interaction was that, not only didn't she feel the need or the right to access the criminal justice system, but that she did, in fact, report the incident to her employer and no law enforcement action was deemed necessary.

To make things even worse, due to a general misunderstanding of HIPAA and other laws governing patient confidentiality, she did not feel that she was able to notify the police. She also told the officer that all her previous training as a nurse caused her to accept that "these things just happen" and that they must be accepted as "part of the job". She also believed that, if she were to pursue an investigation of the incident, it was quite possible she would lose her job.

In her interpretation of her role as a provider, she believed there was actually no recourse for her as a victim. In her mind her position as a provider denied her access to the criminal justice system and even a reasonable expectation of safety. There was no system in place, set by the employer, to protect her from any future occurrence. Instead, there was a professional culture to protect the offender from prosecution. Obviously, the environment of care in which she was working was compatible with violence; furthermore, her acceptance of risk for violent behavior was an expectation of employment. Is that reasonable?

Before we even begin to consider our rights under the law, our beliefs should always be subjected to the smell test of reasonable expectation. It's time to ask ourselves, would she have adopted the above belief system if she were a waitress or a police officer? The answer seems obvious, doesn't it? Then why is it okay to sexually assault a healthcare provider? If she asked a peer or her boss, if this was an acceptable risk, perhaps they might have answered yes. But, what if she asked her mother or her husband? What would any of their perceptions have been? In all likelihood they wouldn't have been as accepting as someone who works in the healthcare field.

This scenario and many like it also begs the question, what if her attacker had just been a visitor or a relative of her patient? What if he had been a fellow employee or just some courier delivering a package to the clinic? The relationship between patient and provider is special, but is culpability for violent behavior really just a matter of context? Do any solid lines exist that no one may cross in the patient-provider relationship? That blurry line is at the heart of the problem of violence in healthcare. *Providers cannot begin to protect themselves from violence in their profession, if they first cannot agree that they are entitled to their own personal safety and basic human dignity.*

Another issue that combines to create a violent culture in healthcare is a lack of basic assessment skills. Though providers are adept at assessing their patient's medical needs, they are generally poor at recognizing the cycle of violence. When we drive a car we look ahead, to the sides and occasionally behind us. We listen, we interpret traffic patterns, we look for danger, and we plan how to extract ourselves from danger. We also think about what measures we might take should danger spontaneously present itself.

Healthcare workers are an entirely different animal. Because they see so many sick and injured people, including many in crisis, they are desensitized to violence. Also, in order to function, they have to work comfortably inside what we normally view as personal space. Because they see us naked, jam needles in us, touch us in very private places, and see people often in varying states of fear and pain, they begin to disregard the pre-attack indicators of violence.

Everyone in a hospital is familiar with the concept of isolation. In order to keep themselves and their patients safe from infection, providers utilize different layers of personal protective gear, facilities, and procedures depending on the situation. For example, if the patient presents with a respiratory infection, the first layers of personal protection are a facemask, gloves, and gown. If more serious infections are suspected, negative pressure isolation rooms, goggles, and other measures are introduced. In this present age of Ebola and MERS, full isolation suits, Tyvek "space suits", filtered air ventilators and even SCBA (self-contained breathing apparatus) may be called for.

It all begins with an assessment. An assessment that answers this question: "How much danger am I in?" What healthcare workers have to begin to embrace is the notion of "forensic isolation." That's because providers are far more frequently hurt or killed by violent patients and visitors than they are by infections resulting from patient care.

Partly due to the extremely large levels of violence experienced by healthcare workers, an entire mythology concerning violence has taken root in the field of medicine. Healthcare has developed a culture of denial — a culture that dismisses threatening and even violent behavior. Healthcare has become, with all well-meaning intentions, a culture that has failed to understand the negative impact of anti-social, uncooperative, threatening, and violent behavior. It is a culture that also fails to understand the influence of unfettered violence on the outcomes of patient care and the well being of healthcare providers.

Gavin de Becker, author of *The Gift of Fear: Survival Signals That Protect Us from Violence*, put it this way, "Only human beings can look directly at something, have all the information they need to make an accurate prediction, perhaps even momentarily make the accurate prediction, and then say that it isn't so." He was referring to a unique feature of the human psyche that causes us to ignore our own instincts. They are the very same instincts that cause a deer to run when it sees a bear in the woods. But when a human being sees a bear, while driving through some National Park, he sometimes gets out of his car and takes a picture. Even though people receive the same danger signals and feel the same fear as a deer, they often disregard them. Sometimes we get the picture we want and other times we get mauled to death. We are the only animals on earth to take such risks for such little return.

That is a great irony considering that we occupy the top of the food chain. Didn't we get to the top partly because of our big brains? Perhaps the ability to rationalize away our fear is why we ride motorcycles, skydive, cross oceans in wooden boats, build skyscrapers, and fly to the moon. On some level, our fearlessness has broadened our experience, enriched our lives, and carried us to horizons other species aren't even capable of imagining. But it is also the same fearlessness that carries us off to war, generation after generation. It is also partly to blame for why, day in and day out, we continually create professional relationships and foster environments of care that are compatible with violence. The purpose of this book is to proclaim that it doesn't have to be that way.

The paradigm of acceptance for violence in healthcare must be abandoned. We must create environments of care and professional relationships that are incompatible with violence and more compatible with patient compliance, cooperation and collaboration.

In any environment, even in a church or a toy store, violence may occur. Still, everyone intuitively understands that some environments are more compatible with violence than others. That notion simply acknowledges that fights are more likely to break out at the corner tavern than your local library — we all get that. Ultimately, the amount of violence that occurs in any setting depends on its established *Social Contract*.

Proper policies, procedures, and training can establish and maintain a *Social Contract* that excludes violence, generates patient collaboration, supports more peaceful and attractive environments of care, and results in better patient outcomes. It all starts with healthcare professionals believing and expecting that violence is unacceptable. Only when healthcare providers embrace a new belief system about violence, can they begin to form safer and more therapeutic relationships with their patients.

Once we've convinced healthcare professionals to stop accepting violence as the norm, we will have to expand their definition of violence. In 2007, Dr. Lauretta Luck, the principle investigator who conducted the seminal *STAMP* study at the University of Western Australia, published her findings in the "Journal of Advanced Nursing," entitled, *STAMP: components of observable behavior that indicate potential for patient violence in emergency departments.* Dr. Luck and her colleagues discovered definite signs in patient and family behavior that reliably signal the potential for violent assaults. Her team organized these behaviors into five categories: staring and eye contact, tone and volume of voice, anxiety, mumbling and pacing.

In most cases, like when sitting on a subway train for instance, we quickly and accurately identify the threatening individuals that might cause us to get up and walk to another seat or get off at the next stop. They are the ones who are staring at us or perhaps looking around in an odd manner. Or perhaps they are talking loudly to another person in an angry tone. They might be rocking back and forth anxiously in their seat. They might be talking to themselves or pacing up and down the aisle. All the above behaviors are familiar signals that this is a person under stress or in crisis. All of them are *STAMP behaviors.* The trouble seems to be that we take action or don't take action, depending solely on the context.

One of the things medical workers often say after a violent assault is, "it happened out of the blue!" That is almost never the case. *In most cases, attackers signal their victims several times that an attack is possible, well before it happens.* This phenomenon is no doubt a function of denial, but the problem may be even worse in healthcare, due to the erosion of our perception of personal space. The concept of *Proxemics 10-5-2*, developed by Dave Young, a Director at Vistelar, are discussed later. These skills are designed to compensate for our lack of healthy fear, as healthcare professionals, and protect us from our own very human impulses to rush in, get to close, and say too much when people are angry and distressed.

STAMP behaviors are no doubt increased in an environment filled with sick, injured, and worried people. That said, it is all the more reason to re-sensitize providers to recognize the *Gateway Behaviors of Violence* and train them how to respond when *STAMP* behaviors are observed. By teaching providers how to respond correctly to behaviors, we can keep them safer.

STAMP behaviors are a kind of gateway behavior. But gateway behaviors can also be very deliberate. When someone begins to curse, for instance, in an environment where it would commonly be viewed as inappropriate, they are often trying to elicit a response from bystanders. When persons curse in front of children and families in our hospitals and clinics and we say nothing, the non-verbal messages of our silence are "it's acceptable", "I'm afraid", "I have no authority" or "I don't care."

When people curse and otherwise behave inappropriately, they are sending out, what are in a sense, verbal "radar waves" to see what signals bounce back. When the answer they receive is silence, they begin to gain power and authority over the group. Once they become comfortable with making others uncomfortable, they begin to turn up the heat. Often this takes the form of yelling or shouting. When we remain silent they also become comfortable shouting at us. Then they begin to threaten us, often in the form of an implied or veiled threat. Examples are, "Touch my kid again and see what happens" or "Send that doctor in here again and she'll be sorry."

Once people become comfortable implying they will hurt us, then they often just blatantly threaten us, by saying things like "Stick me one more time and I'll knock you out!" *In healthcare, perhaps more than in any other profession, customers routinely threaten staff with absolute impunity.* So, when people get comfortable threatening us and they can do so with impunity, why not hit us? That is the question we often place in the minds of our attackers, when we fail to train to manage aggression and set limits on bad behavior. All cycles of interpersonal violence develop this way, whether it's one between nations or individuals. Whether it's a schoolyard fight or a domestic violence relationship, it all begins the same way and usually ends up badly for the victim.

When gateway behaviors are observed in patients and visitors, trained healthcare providers can reliably minimize their anxiety, assuage their fear, set limits on inappropriate behaviors, and address their underlying issues, thereby diffusing the potential for violence. That formula leads to safer and better medicine. People get better medicine because, if people feel safe in our hospitals and clinics, they might not avoid them. Also, if healthcare providers don't fear their patients or their visitors, they might spend more time with them and make fewer mistakes.

If we intervene early in the gateway behavior cycle, we can stop the journey towards violence. If we can stop people from cursing and yelling, they may not graduate to threatening and violent behavior. Ultimately, it is much easier to stop someone from yelling than it is to stop them from hitting. But we can't even begin, if we don't understand how or when.

Even in the most peaceful environment, anyone can find themselves in a threatening or violent situation. No violence prevention and management system would be complete, unless we trained providers and staff what to do to diffuse violence, should it rear its ugly head. Everyone understands that before we can learn to run, we must first learn to walk. So doesn't it stand to reason that before we learn to de-escalate, we should learn to *non-escalate?* The concept of *non-escalation* is a cornerstone of what we do as healthcare violence consultants and trainers at Vistelar and is part and parcel of creating environments of care that are incompatible with violence.

If you still doubt that focusing on unwanted behaviors can lead to systemic change, you might consider this. When I began my career in healthcare in 1991, smoking was allowed in hospitals. Scarcely a decade ago smoking was pushed completely outside of American hospitals, as their ever-shrinking "smoking lounges" were closed down and smokers were banished to the sidewalk. Now smoking isn't even allowed on most hospital campuses.

Restaurants no longer allow smoking, despite all the unfounded fears of restaurant owners that their businesses would close down. Then soon followed the bars and taverns; the last vestige of public smoking, the places where nobody thought smoking would ever fade away. Now you can't rent a hotel room or even an apartment that allows smoking by its tenants. In a few short years we, as a society, decided to address smoking; and, as a result we have all but driven smoking entirely from the public experience. Something many speculated could never be done.

Joel Lashley

Chapter Two
Everything Is Okay Now
Respond, Don't React

"Violence can only be concealed by a lie, and the lie can only be maintained by violence."

Aleksandr Solzhenitsyn

The security team arrived on the unit in just a few minutes, but the floor was already quiet. The call from dispatch said a nurse was being actively assaulted, so everyone double-timed it up to the floor. When they arrived at the patient's room, the door was closed and they were silently greeted by a doctor and some nurses standing outside. Andrea, the first arriving officer, was also the first to break the silence. "Is everyone okay? What happened?" she asked.

"Everything is okay now," replied the doctor.

"Well that's a relief," replied Andrea. "Is anyone hurt?"

To that, the doctor looked sufficiently annoyed and replied, "Nope. It was just a little misunderstanding. Everything is fine now, so you can all go back to work."

"Can I at least see the nurse who said she was assaulted? I have a report to write," replied Andrea, as she stepped toward the patient's room.

"Is that really necessary?" he said and stepped in front of her.

Concealed inside the room was the startled patient, curled up in her bed, as her nurse lay unconscious on the floor. The visitor who had struck the nurse had fled down a stairwell, just seconds before the security team had arrived. Oblivious to the medical emergency behind him, the doctor continued to argue with the security team, while precious minutes flew by, saying "If you go in there you will only make things worse."

In his defense, the doctor had no idea the extent of the injuries to the nurse, having arrived just a few seconds prior to the security team. He hadn't witnessed the assault but was told by the nurses on the unit that there was a fight in his patient's room. At that moment, he was only operating on a flawed but very common instinct among providers. That instinct was to advocate for his patient, no matter what the circumstances. In his eyes, keeping security and the hospital's administration out of the provider-patient relationship was his first priority.

If he had been trained in the *First Responder Philosophy (FRP)*, his first instincts after he'd arrived would have been to assess the scene by listening, by looking and by quickly asking questions of the nursing staff. Then he would have raised the alarm by calling for security himself. Luckily, someone who was thinking more clearly had already done that. His next step would have been to evaluate the scene to determine if it was safe for him to enter the room alone or wait for the security team.

Then he and/or the security team would enter the room where they would have seen the nurse unconscious on the floor. Their next step would have been to stabilize the scene. Although the perpetrator had already fled, an injured nurse and a frightened patient both needed care. So the physician could have started the next step—an initial medical assessment of the unconscious nurse while other nurses saw to the patient's needs.

The *First Responder Philosophy* then would have also triggered the long-term monitoring phase, where the physician would have called for a medical response team to transport the nurse to the emergency department for further treatment. The next step would involve communication between the security team, the police, and hospital administration so the suspect could be apprehended, searched and identified. Finally, the *FRP* would require that all parties document and debrief the incident, so a risk assessment could be completed, and a safety plan implemented to protect everyone from future risk.

The *First Responder Philosophy* has a long history of improving institutional responses in everything from hospitals to prisons. It safely and effectively guides teams to manage incidents involving fire, medical emergencies, violent disturbances, and miscellaneous incidents, like chemical spills and utility shutdowns.

Since I was first trained to use the *FRP* in a hospital setting over two decades ago, I have relied on it. It was developed by Gary Klugiewicz, Bob Willis and their colleagues for the State of Wisconsin Department of Corrections. If the physician of our story had been trained in the *First Responder Philosophy*, things probably would have gone very differently when he'd first arrived on the scene.

Aside from a lack of training in a response model like the *First Responder Philosophy*, what else might have caused the disconnection between the medical staff, the security staff, and, ultimately, the hospital administration in this instance? Perhaps it was the overall acceptance of violence in healthcare. Certainly, the doctor wouldn't have barred access to the patient's room, if the smell of smoke was wafting from the room. Yet, both nurses and patients are injured by violence with far more regularity than fire. Perhaps healthcare professionals must begin to understand that violence is an institutional emergency, just like a fire, flood, or a power outage.

If you still don't agree that the acceptance of violence in healthcare is one of the cultural drivers that lead us along a path of endemic violence, consider the many general myths people commonly embrace about violence (e.g., "bullying toughens kids up;" "always smile when dealing with the public"). In this book we'll discuss seven violence-enabling myths that are prevalent in healthcare.

Myth #1: "If you say something, it will make things worse."

This one tops the list for me. It's the myth I hear most often and perhaps the one that does the most damage. If you've worked in healthcare for even a short while, you've probably heard this one. Worse yet, you've probably come to embrace it on some level. So, if you've heard this myth, forget it. And, if you hear someone say it, correct them.

The fact is, if we ask someone confidently and respectfully to stop behaving badly, they usually will comply. When we say nothing, while people behave badly in our presence, the non-verbal messages of silence are permission and submission. Specifically, if we say nothing when people threaten or even demean us, the non-verbal messages are, "it's okay to behave that way" or "I have no authority to act." Perhaps, the worst of all nonverbal messages is, "I'm afraid." Failing to speak up when people need limits set on bad behavior usually ensures that we'll get more bad behavior and that it will escalate.

If the people involved in the angry biker situation had believed this myth, no one would have addressed his behavior, and certainly not with any consistency. What also can be learned from the angry biker is that, *if we focus on behavior, the attitude will follow.* That is another important principle for establishing a therapeutic relationship. Skilled communicators focus on a person's behavior, not their attitude. What we do naturally is to focus on a person's attitude hoping that their behavior will improve. This rarely works and even backfires as the aggressor feels empowered by your attempts to assuage their anger, by incessant apologies, by allowing them to vent, and by otherwise rewarding their bad behaviors. To make things worse, if all you've been trained to do is service recovery and/or crisis intervention, then appeasement is probably the only skill you've ever been taught.

Myth #2: "Don't sweat the small stuff."

Another reason there is so much violence in healthcare is because our definition of violence is too narrow. As already stated, everyone knows not to drop f-bombs in church or talk loudly in a library. But why do so many people yell, curse and threaten in a hospital? Is it simply because some people behave badly when they're sick? Or is it because they believe they are *entitled* to behave badly, simply because they're sick? Perhaps it's because healthcare workers believe patients have a right to behave badly. In reality, it's all the above.

Once we've decided to set limits on bad behaviors, we'll all be safer. But if we set the bar too low, we'll often end up acting too late. In healthcare, we have to remind ourselves that nice people don't hurt us — angry, anti-social, and threatening people do! Because behaviors are connected, people usually build up to violence. They start with refusing to follow visiting hours, refusing to wear visitors' passes, cursing, yelling or threatening, well before they attack. If we start to set limits when people first begin to violate our *Social Contract,* they are more likely to become cooperative and less likely to become violent.

Myth #3: "Kill them with kindness"

This is the myth that goes like this, "Just be nice when people abuse you, because if you're real nice to them, they will start to like you and stop abusing you." I call this the myth of submission. Submission is a survival skill. It's a natural tactic for finding a place in the pecking order of nature. When we behave this way we are telling the person who is behaving badly that they are in charge and that we're afraid. We can't answer bad behavior with more bad behavior, so it's not about challenging the aggressor. It's about setting the appropriate *Social Contract* and maintaining it.

Without going into too much detail about this myth, its efficacy can be tested with a question: Would you tell someone involved in a domestic violence relationship to kill their tormentor with kindness? If your sister or daughter told you that their husband or boyfriend was abusing them, would you tell her to just fix herself up and be more romantic? Would you tell her to shower her man with love and attention? Of course you wouldn't. Then why do we keep giving each other essentially the same bad advice in healthcare?

Myth #4: "People behave badly because they are sick and under stress."

Is this really true? Cumulatively, I've spent hundreds of days of my life in acute care as a consumer. I once spent a month in a hospital recovering from a painful and complex orthopedic surgery. My son has had five operations in total. My father had several cancers, before liver cancer finally took him. My late wife had a twenty-year long chronic and severe health condition, before it finally took her. In all that time, through all that stress, fear and pain, I never yelled at, cursed at, or threatened a healthcare provider.

Does that make me special? Absolutely not! In fact, the majority of people who visit our clinics and hospitals everyday never threaten us or otherwise behave inappropriately. It's only a small number of people who make the healthcare environment uncomfortable and unsafe. Sure, perhaps people are more likely to act out when under stress. No one wants to be in a hospital. Everyone there is either sick or connected to someone who is. That said, if we set limits on behaviors effectively and provide the kind of support that people in crisis really need, then we can have more peaceful and therapeutic environments of care for everyone.

Myth #5: "Violence is just part of the job."

We've got to stop saying this, because this myth is literally killing us. I've heard this one since the first day I started working in healthcare in 1991. Just like in any other cycle of violence, if we accept this myth, we are paralyzed to act and doomed to remain victims. Because so many people embrace this myth, the majority of schools are unsafe for many children who find themselves endlessly bullied and hopeless. Because of this myth, residents and staff of group homes for people with psychiatric conditions and brain-based disorders are commonly locked in a daily cycle of violence and fear. And staff are assaulted on the job at rates at least seven times more than average.

Why is it that if a nurse threatened a patient we would fire him or her without question? But when a patient threatens, shoves, spits at, and perhaps even slaps a provider, we are hesitant to even call security? It's partly because of this pervasive and destructive myth. Abraham Lincoln once said, "Familiarize yourselves with the chains of bondage and you prepare your own limbs to wear them." His point was that if all are not free then none of us are assured of our freedom. Likewise, just as we must ensure the safety of our patients we must ensure the safety of our providers. But we'll never get to a safer place in healthcare until we can at least agree that a safer place exists!

If we can't eliminate disrespect and fear for healthcare providers, then we cannot eliminate them for our patients either. Peggy Troy, the CEO of Children's Hospital of Wisconsin, is fond of saying "The patient experience cannot surpass the employee experience."

She understands the experience of the patient and the provider are inextricably bound together. Unfettered anti-social behavior not only leads to violence, but it sours the environment of care for everyone—staff and patients alike.

Myth #6: "The Customer is Always Right"

Almost one in three surveyed emergency department and family practice physicians has admitted to prescribing antibiotics to patients who didn't need them, even though everyone knows the overuse of antibiotics is a threat to public health! Even more shocking, two out of three surveyed doctors have admitted to delaying vaccines in pediatric patients due to unscientific and misguided beliefs embraced by their parents. Sadly, most of them did so knowing full well that it was unhealthy for their patients and for public health. As a result, the CDC fears that measles and whooping cough are back with a vengeance and probably more resurgences of dangerous diseases in children are yet to come. Why? The reason most often given by physicians was pressure from their patient's parents.

Somewhere along the line, we started treating healthcare like retail and not as a profession of higher calling. Yes it's a competitive environment, but where do we draw the line? I propose the line exists where unscientific notions impinge on the interests of patient care and public health. Perhaps we can start by ceasing to view patients as merely customers. The "customer" isn't right when they impinge on the rights of others. And, if the "customer" is endangering their own health or that of others by acting against medical advice, providers have to persuade and educate them. But that takes training and a new way of doing business.

The best place to start is to rediscover our professionalism in healthcare. A hospital is not a department store. It is an institution of healing and education. If so many doctors are failing to influence the healthcare decisions of their patients, then perhaps communications training, and not crisis intervention theory, is the answer.

Myth #7: "Things really aren't that bad."

Once while I was waiting to meet with a physician and his staff about a patient who had threatened his life, I struck up a conversation with one of his nurses. I asked her if anything like this had ever happened before. She said it hadn't and that she was in shock over the whole incident. Nonetheless, she thought the whole thing was silly and that the doctor was making way too much of things.

I then asked her how long she'd been in nursing. She explained she'd been a nurse for more than 30 years and worked in many specialties, as an RN and Master Degree prepared nurse. I then asked her if she'd experienced much violence on the job. She replied, "Not really. Things really aren't that bad. A little conflict here and there is just part of the job." I then asked her if a patient or visitor had ever shoved her, and she said "sure." I then asked her if anyone had ever slapped her and she said, "I've been slapped a couple times, sure." I asked her if she'd ever been kicked, punched, grabbed, or spit on and she answered yes to all. Finally, I asked her what sort of behavior did she consider to be violent. She replied, "Yeah, I see where you're going, but I used to be an E.R. nurse. A lot of that stuff happened there. After that, I would only get attacked by someone once in a blue moon."

As previously stated, if you work as nurse in a hospital, you are at least five times more likely to be physically assaulted than the average wage-earner and if you work in an emergency department, that number at least doubles. We need to act now. It's time to ask ourselves if this is really the way it has to be. Are we getting anywhere by denying there's a problem? Are we getting any safer? Have our notions of family-centered care and the old methods of crisis prevention even made a dent or are they propagating and perpetuating the very same mythology that keeps us locked in a cycle of violence? So what is the solution? Perhaps one can be found among the seven answers to the seven myths of violence in healthcare.

All of the skill sets described in this book are intended to develop a pre-planned, practiced, response in the practitioner, so that they can successfully manage conflict and treat their patients. In order for them to be successful, the institutions they work in must support them by creating an environment of care that is incompatible with anti-social and violent behavior. In answer to the seven myths, the following seven steps prepare a hospital or clinic to begin constructing a safer and more therapeutic environment.

Step #1: Create the expectation that everyone must *Take Appropriate Action* whenever anti-social and violent behavior is observed.

Healthcare workers have to adopt a *"hear something — do something"* mentality when it comes to violence. They must be trained to consistently address the *Gateway Behaviors of Violence* when they see and hear them, then *Take Appropriate Action*. They also must learn to judge whether to take action with their co-workers and when it's necessary to call security or law enforcement. The concept of *when word-based tactics fail* will be discussed in a later chapter.

Step #2: Adopt a clear and broad definition of violence.

Because violent behavior is connected through gateway behaviors, we need to include anti-social and threatening behaviors in our definition of violence. Also the refusal to follow basic policies and procedures by patients and visitors should not go unnoticed and unanswered, even if we don't directly identify such resistance as violent behavior. If we can't get someone to comply with something as seemingly insignificant as wearing a visitor' pass, then how do we expect to persuade them to cooperate when the stakes are even higher?

At the very least, a clear definition of inappropriate and violent behavior in a hospital should always include behaviors that disturb or offend others, such as: demeaning language or comments regarding a person's race, religion, sexual orientation, age, body shape; profanity, swearing or cursing; shouting, yelling, or loud talking; implied or overt verbal threats; sexual comments and unwanted advances; touching without permission (unless necessary for the safety of self or others); behavior that disturbs others or causes fear, in patients, visitors, and staff.

Step #3: Train providers and staff to perform non-escalation skills.

Non-escalation is a unique skill set that practitioners of Vistelar's conflict management methodologies practice and learn in scenario-based drills. Gary Klugiewicz, a Director at Vistelar, often says, "The best way to avoid a fight is to never start the negative dance." By training everyone according to the five approaches to showing respect, *the Showtime Mindset,* and the *Universal Greeting* (all discussed in later chapters), we can begin to establish an environment of care that is incompatible with anti-social behavior and violence.

Step #4: Train providers and staff to perform de-escalation skills.

Whether we like it or not just about everyone who walks into a hospital doesn't want to be there. Most people walk in the front door with four or five problems. They are sick or someone they love is sick. They are missing time from work. They don't have insurance or have high deductibles. Their spouse is unsupportive when they are sick or when one of the kids is sick. Some have other kids at home that need their attention. So many other possible stressors can pile on top of a hospitalization: pain, fear, health problems, financial problems, relationship problems and professional problems.

Little wonder there is a lot of violence in healthcare, but the potential for violence exists in many other professions as well, such as prison work and even banking. All these issues are just part of the picture, but they are a significant part. By training staff to recognize the signs of crisis, pre-attack postures, *STAMP* and gateway behaviors, we can arm them to make on the spot safety assessments and "change gears" in their approach.

For example, in Vistelar's *Point of Impact Crisis Intervention* program students are taught to reduce stimulation, separate and support, adapt communication, and manage unmet needs—quickly and safely in order to de-escalate people in crisis. Untrained or insufficiently trained people tend to do what comes natural when they attempt to de-escalate people in crisis. And what they naturally do is get too close, talk too loud, and say too much.

Step #5: Adopt a zero-tolerance policy for violence and clearly define zero-tolerance.

Zero-tolerance does not mean that we throw everybody out who yells or curses in a hospital. It does require that we consistently address issues, like cursing and yelling, when they are first observed. If we can't effectively and reasonably reign in uncooperative, anti-therapeutic, and anti-social behavior, then clear consequences have to be presented and enforced. When we are threatened or attacked, those consequences have to include loss of visitation rights and police involvement. In some cases it will even require refusal of service to patients. Healthcare is the only profession I know of where its customers can threaten or even assault workers with impunity. That has to change.

That said, people in crisis behave badly sometimes. First we must start by teaching staff to recognize crisis behaviors and distinguish them from anti-social behaviors. People in genuine crisis, who are yelling and otherwise acting-out may be reacting to medication, bad news, pain, and psychiatric conditions. These patients need privacy and support. Nonetheless, violent assaults generally should be reported to the police, even when they are the result of a crisis. The medical profession will become a lot safer when it more effectively partners with the law enforcement profession to determine criminality. The determination about whether criminal charges are appropriate are best determined after an investigation, not at the point of impact.

Injuries often occur when patients are in altered states of consciousness, such as when coming out of anesthesia. Many other patients suffer from brain injuries and brain-based disorders that can cause them to act-out. Healthcare workers must be trained to recognize, safely stabilize, and disengage from acting-out patients—and, if they are, fewer injuries will occur. In a recent *Interventions for Patients with Challenging Behaviors* course, a nursing supervisor said, "If I had known these skills last week, one of my nurses wouldn't have been injured. I'm certain of it. I would have known what to do to keep us safe." Just a couple of weeks after that, she was able to fulfill that prediction, as she reportedly led her team to safely stabilize a violent patient on her unit. Fortunately, this time no one was injured, including the patient.

Step #6: Train to persuade and educate patients in evidence-based practices.

Another one of the core skills discussed in this book is the *Persuasion Sequence*, which is founded on Vistelar's five approaches to showing respect (covered in the next chapter). Just as with the angry biker, medical workers can use it to persuade patients to cooperate and even collaborate with proper medical care.

First, clinicians are trained to ask someone to cooperate, in a confident and professional tone of voice, while wearing the appropriate expression. Then they are trained how to set context, or explain why it's in their interest to accept sound medical advice.

When done well, most patients will cooperate. If not, students of Vistelar's conflict management methodologies are trained to *offer choices or present options*. When providers effectively help their patients to understand the benefits of recommended therapy versus the dangers of inaction, most patients will choose the right option.

It takes training and practice to lock-down context for uncooperative or fearful patients and loved ones, but it can be done reliably by trained communicators. For those patients who still refuse to cooperate, providers can confirm their intentions by offering them another chance to comply. When unsuccessful, providers have to be clear on their limits. No provider should ever prescribe a drug they know might be harmful to a patient. And when patients behave in a way that is detrimental to their health and the health of others, providers must be willing to *Take Appropriate Action*, up to and including discharging them from their practice.

Step #7: Make clear to everyone their right to protect themselves and their responsibility to protect patients in their care.

Many human service workers honestly believe they do not have the right to protect themselves or their clients, because they've been told throughout their career to never touch a client without permission— no matter what the circumstances! This belief is obvious nonsense to some healthcare professionals, but it's an absolute truth to others.

The right to self-protection is an inalienable human right and no state can make a law taking away the right to self-protection. Although many institutions have flirted with the issue, no hospital, nursing facility, group home or other employer can enforce a policy that infringes on an individual's right to self-defense, anymore than they can ask them not to breathe! Also, no one can avoid the responsibility to protect patients in their care. Sometimes that means going hands-on. What should medical workers do if their patient is about to swallow a bottle of pills, just watch? Ask some medical workers that question and you may get some surprising answers.

Many people, who work outside the healthcare field, would be shocked to learn how little training nurses receive in even the most basic stabilization skills, such as stabilizing a combative patient in the supine position. And that's despite the fact that more injuries result from combative patients than from errant needle sticks! Therefore, due to the alarming rates of violence in hospitals and the responsibility for healthcare workers to care for people in distress, it is an absolute necessity to train medical workers in basic self-protection and stabilization skills.

Joel Lashley

Chapter Three
Visiting Hours Are Over
Showing Respect, Showtime Mindset

"An eye for an eye will make the whole world blind."

Mahatma Gandhi

In my career I've worked in several healthcare facilities, including everything from large urban hospitals to sub-acute centers located in the heart of street gang territory. Many years ago when I was training for a job as a hospital security officer, I was shadowing another officer to learn the procedures at a visitors' desk.

Our assignment was to greet everyone attempting to enter the main entrance to the hospital, after visiting hours had ended. We were to determine why they were there, give them a visitor's pass, and direct them to their destination when appropriate. That part was easy. The difficult part came when we had to tell people that only immediate family were allowed to visit after hours and that they couldn't visit their neighbor, co-worker, or nephew. As you can imagine, no one was ever happy to get that news.

When visiting hours ended at 8PM, my training officer and I

locked all the front doors except for one. Then we put out the sign, turned down the lights, took our seats, and waited. We didn't have to wait long. By 8:15 the first would-be visitor walked right past the "Visiting Hours Are Over" sign and up to the visiting center. My training officer took the lead as it was my first day on the job. The officer greeted the visitor by simply stating, "Welcome to the General Hospital, how can I help you?"

"I'm here to visit somebody," began the visitor.

"Okay, how are you related?" asked my training officer in a somber tone of voice.

"Uh, well, I'm not. She's just a friend," replied the young man.

The officer replied, "Visiting hours are over."

After a pregnant pause, during which the two men stared blankly at each other, the visitor replied, "Really? Can I just run up and say hi for a second?"

The officer looked up at the man and replied in a disinterested tone, "Well, visiting hours are over, so you'll have to come back tomorrow."

"That's ridiculous," replied the man.

"Sorry but that's the way it is. I don't make the rules," said the officer.

"Well you don't have to be a jerk about it!" fired back the man in an angry tone of voice.

After a little more back and forth, the conversation deteriorated into a shouting match. The man left in a huff, while threatening to call and complain about what he believed was the shabby way he'd been treated. Now sitting in silence, I could tell that this was not my training officer's favorite part of the job.

By 8:30, another visitor arrived. A high-energy middle-aged woman appeared at our desk, beaming a broad smile and carrying a grocery bag full of treats, magazines, and toiletries for some hapless patient. Seeming to notice my training officer's blank expression and lack of eye contact, she took a couple of steps over to address me instead.

"Hello. Welcome to General Hospital. How can I help you this evening?" I said.

"I need to get to the maternity ward. My neighbor is having a baby and she forgot some things at home. This is such an exciting time! It's her first baby!" she said.

"Well how nice of you to bring her things down…" I began to say before being interrupted by my training officer.

The officer leaned over and blurted in a terse tone, "Sorry, but visiting hours are over."

The woman nervously blinked, wearing an expression of surprised disappointment, and said, "Oh poo. Can I just run these things up to her? She has no clothes or anything. She's waiting for them."

"You'll have to come back tomorrow. They have anything she will need up on the floor," said the officer.

The woman's expression went from disappointment to indignation. "Well, she said I could bring these things down. Could someone at least take them up to her?"

"We really don't have anyone available to do that," he replied, wearing his signature expression of disinterest.

"Then can I leave them here until someone is available to run them up to her?" she retorted angrily.

"We can't accept things from visitors. We can't be responsible for them," he fired back.

"I want to talk to your supervisor, this is ridiculous!" she replied tersely.

At that point the officer did as trained and called the charge nurse on the unit. She instructed the officer to issue a visitor's pass and send the woman up. With a look of satisfaction, the woman took her pass and walked toward the elevators that would take her to the obstetrics floor. "See that?" he asked me. "Sometimes it doesn't even pay to try and stop anyone from visiting."

A few minutes later, a young couple and their two young children approached the desk. The kids were holding balloons and smiling happily in anticipation of visiting their cousin in the hospital. This time I stayed silent and waited for my training officer to begin. He looked down at his desk with a look of obvious frustration and said, "Welcome to General Hospital. How can I help you?"

"We need to go to pediatrics," replied the woman in a pleasant tone of voice.

"How are you related to the patient, Ma'am?"

"He's our nephew and these are his cousins" she replied pleasantly, while motioning towards her smiling and well-behaved children.

"Only immediate family after eight o'clock. I'm sorry," he replied tersely, clearly frustrated by a bad start to the evening.

As you can imagine, the conversation went south from there. After a couple more exchanges, the security supervisor was called to the desk to deal with the angry couple. Soon after the supervisor and the disappointed family left, my training officer looked over at me and said in frustration, "Boy, people are sure showing up in a crappy mood tonight."

The main thing I learned from that training officer on my first day was how not to communicate with patients and visitors. As the evening went on, every visitor who was turned away seemed to leave with a bad impression. They not only left with a bad impression of my training officer, but of me as well. They also left with a bad impression of the hospital, as we were both guilty by association.

Healthcare is a high-stakes profession. Just as in law enforcement, many of the daily decisions that healthcare workers make can drastically affect the lives of the people they serve. If we accept that as true, then a professional's outlook—whether they are a police officer, a teacher, or a doctor—should be such that it best serves the interest of the people who place their trust in them. That said, the routine of human service work—where professionals frequently encounter people at their most anxious, angry, or defiant—challenges the professional's positive outlook toward the people they serve. As a result, human service professionals often develop a negative mind set towards their clients.

Criminal Justice educators and trainers sometimes refer to the *90/10 Ratio* in law enforcement. The *90/10 Ratio* refers to the belief that 90 percent of the people in the world are basically good and ten percent are basically bad. While most of us (the ninety percent) obey the law and contribute positively in some way to society, a smaller number of people (represented by a figure of ten percent) are responsible for most of the conflict, crime, and iniquity in the world. However, some law enforcement professionals believe that, due to daily exposures to people behaving badly, many officers flip the 90/10 ratio over to a 10/90 ratio—a point of view in which the law enforcement officer believes that only ten percent of the world is filled with good people, meaning that 9 out of 10 people are jerks, law breakers, and untrustworthy.

The *10/90 Ratio* outlook is one that healthcare professionals often fall victim to as well. If that's the case, could the belief that most of the people who walk into our emergency rooms and clinics are bad people negatively affect our interactions with patients at the point of impact? The concept is at least worth exploring.

As I worked over the next few weeks with that training officer as my guide, I learned a great deal about him. He could, in fact, be a very personable guy. He was well liked by his co-workers in the security department. The nursing staff in the emergency room liked him as well. He was funny and friendly. He got along well with everyone it seemed, except ironically, the people whom we were there to serve. He was poor with his communication at the welcome centers, on the floor, or anywhere else that he was called upon to deal with patients and families. After working alongside him for a while, I started to build an understanding of why he struggled to communicate with the hospital's customers.

Armed with the supposition that anyone who walked past a sign that read "Visiting Hours Are Over" is either a jerk or stupid, he greeted them all with an annoyed expression and a disinterested tone. He visibly avoided eye contact with people as they approached the desk, instead looking down at his computer screen, at the counter top, or over at me. When a visitor approached the welcome center, he would offer his canned greeting of "Welcome to General Hospital, how can I help you?" at a fast pace and in a monotone voice. When challenged, he would offer no explanations, no solutions, no empathy, and no regret. He would offer none of these things with his words, with his tone or volume of voice, or even with the expression of his face.

When dealing with disturbance calls on a nursing unit, or anywhere else in the hospital, he also struggled hopelessly. He rarely got compliance from people and had to rely on supervisors and co-workers to try and bail him out. When on patrol, he often looked the other way when seeing or hearing issues that should be addressed, just to avoid confrontation. Though he obviously was adept at communicating in social situations, he was inept at communicating in the midst of conflict. And he is not alone. Communicating under pressure is difficult for everyone, but it's what we do most often as human service professionals—talk to people under pressure. Still, we spend very little time, if any, learning how to do it.

The first step in learning how to communicate under pressure is to work on the 10/90 mindset—the belief that everyone we deal with is a jerk and that no matter what we say or do, we cannot win when dealing with them. To achieve this mindset change we must begin with a better understanding of human nature.

A core principle Vistelar teaches about human nature is that *everyone deserves to be treated with dignity by showing them respect* and that, to show respect, you must follow these five approaches 1) See the world through their eyes; 2) Listen with all your senses; 3) Ask and explain why; 4) Offer options, let them choose, 5) Give opportunity to reconsider.

One of the best lessons I ever got on treating people with dignity by showing respect was from a co-worker. A manager in an office where I once worked decided to print and post pictures of all the important people in the company. Being a very large company, we ended up with many faces posted on our office wall. Under each of the faces of the CEO, President, many Vice Presidents and department heads, were their names, departments and titles. Almost daily, whenever he walked through our office, he would say, "Now you guys all learn these names and faces. When you see them, show them respect and make sure you are on your best behavior!" Soon, his little "respect" speech became a familiar feature of our office life.

After a few weeks of pounding home the need to respect important people in the company, he started to quiz us. He would catch some unfortunate person walking by his "wall of fame", as he called it, and cover the title section under one of the pictures with his hand. He would then ask, "What's this person's name, department and title?" If we got it right he'd say, "good job." If we got it wrong, we got dressed down. In short, he wasn't treating any of us with much respect. In fact, he had quite a reputation around the company as being a jerk. He wasn't well liked by much of the staff in our department or in any other department. But he was liked, however, by a lot of people in authority. Probably because he practiced what he preached.

If he bumped into someone important, he would smile and greet them in an exuberant and friendly fashion. He would call them by name and complement their clothes or haircut. He would congratulate them on a promotion or tell them how much he appreciated their contribution to the company. His reputation, however, was very different among his own staff and other employees of the company. In fact, he was viewed by many as being unfriendly, demeaning, and rude. Some saw him as racist and sexist, and complaints were not uncommon about his attitude and behavior. Still, he plugged along happily day after day, instructing all of us to treat people with respect, as long as they were someone in authority.

On one particular day, this manager looked around the office and called over another manager to review his "wall of shame", as it had become popularly known. He placed his hand over the title section of one picture and asked the other manager if he knew who that was. The other manager looked around at all of us in the room. On our faces he saw expressions of embarrassment, disgust, and discomfort. Then he looked at the manager and simply said, "You know what? If you would just learn to treat everyone with dignity by showing them respect, you wouldn't have to memorize these names and faces." By the next day, the "wall of shame" was gone. It was taken down and thrown in the wastebasket by some anonymous person and was never put up again.

If my old training officer at the hospital where I once worked had known and embraced Vistelar's five approaches to showing respect, chances are he would have been one step closer to being as successful with the people he served as he was with the people he worked alongside. Although he resisted professional communications training (Verbal Defense & Influence) at first, over-time he embraced it as he saw others using it and succeeding under pressure. Now he is well respected, highly competent, and a hospital security leader. His former weakness had become one of his greatest strengths, as he is often sought out to have difficult conversations in difficult situations. If my old manager, with the "wall of shame", had treated everyone with dignity by showing them respect, and not just the people in charge, he wouldn't have lost his job, which eventually he did. He lost it because of all the disrespect he had shown and the complaints he generated as a result.

Vistelar's five approaches to showing respect are not only the basis for treating people with dignity but for persuading them to cooperate (which you'll learn in a later chapter). But, for the five approaches to be successful, both the words you say and how you say them are critical. That is why it's important to understand and adopt the *Showtime Mindset*.

On another occasion, I was given the assignment of protecting a social worker while she addressed the behavior of a threatening family in a hospital. We were to go to the room of a gravely ill child and readdress the parents recurring threatening language towards staff. The patient was chronically ill, experiencing frequent and lengthy hospitalizations. The parents reportedly fought daily between themselves, and cursing and yelling were regularly heard on the unit. Frequent attempts to rein in their behavior had failed and all involved were at a loss about what to do.

As luck would have it, by the time we arrived on the unit we could already hear yelling and cursing coming from the patient's room. As soon as we arrived at the room, a fearful nurse ran out and scooted quickly down the hallway. Before arriving our roles for the intervention had been clearly defined. The social worker was to do all the talking and I was to observe and protect if necessary. The social worker walked into the room wearing a surprised expression, with me on her heels and remaining silent as asked.

The social worker began by saying in an urgent tone, "Hey, what's all the yelling about?"

"We don't have time for this bulls***," replied the father. As you can imagine, the conversation spiraled out of control. When the father got louder, the social worker shouted back, matching his tone and intensity. When he accused the nursing staff of incompetence and indifference she became defensive. Soon, both the mother and the father were standing and facing off, nose-to-nose with the social worker!

Just as I was about to step in, there was a loud knock on the doorframe. After getting everyone's attention, the Director of Security walked in. Wearing a business suit and an expression that could only be described as a concerned smile, he walked towards the parents with his hand outstretched and said, "Please allow me to introduce myself." At that, the startled parents stood silent. Then suddenly, the father smiled brightly and took the Director's hand, saying, "See, that's how you come into someone's room!"

Simply put, the *Showtime Mindset* refers to the necessity to always be on stage when we're at work. Walt Disney, in all his genius, understood this concept very well. He understood the experience of the customer is always tied to presentation. That's why you'll never see a guy in a Mickey Mouse costume sitting at a lunch counter in Disneyland, with the head of his costume sitting next to him while he eats a hamburger. Disney understood he could never take the chance of revealing to the kids passing by that there is only an ordinary man inside that costume. He also understood that Mickey's little secret was just as important for the adults who visited his theme park. It was Mickey, Goofy, Snow White and all the little characters that set the tone for the experience — not just people inside colorful costumes.

Vistelar's conflict management training takes practitioners through drills that develop their Showtime Mindset. In training, they learn to adapt their non-verbal and verbal communications skills. Habits like nervous smiling, crowding, matching volume, matching tone, and verbal overload are identified and worked on in a way that builds psychomotor skills in the learner. After all, speech and communication is very much a psychomotor skill. Scenario based training in professional communication gives the student the feeling that they've been there before when difficult situations arise. By building these memories in training, we can transfer *canned experience* to the real world. This is something that cannot be achieved in a book or video presentation.

Managers in customer service commonly instruct their employees to smile. "Always wear a smile" is a mantra heard in retail establishments across America and generally it's good advice. I agree that in most circumstances people need to look approachable and friendly while at work, whether they are a police officer, nurse, or cashier. That is an important part of developing a *Showtime Mindset*. But just as with anything else, people need more than one tool on their belt.

Many years after my first day on the job as a hospital security officer, I was working as a communications skills trainer. I was asked by a patient representative department manager to mentor one of her information center employees. At this particular institution, visitation staff, not security officers, staffed the information centers or welcome centers, even after hours. The manager advised me that her employee was struggling in her job and had received several complaints. She wasn't sure why, because the employee was really quite personable, but she would be forced to terminate her if complaints continued to roll in.

When I finally learned the welcome center staff member's name, I was shocked. "Her?" I said, "She's the nicest lady here! Everyone loves her!" This was one of those employees who was always smiling and friendly. She always offered a big "hello" for everyone who walked in the door. She always made an obvious effort to make every patient, visitor and employee feel truly welcome. Frankly, I was stumped. Unbeknownst to her, I watched her work for a few hours and couldn't understand why she was generating so many complaints. On the outside, she appeared to be a master of the *Showtime* persona.

As you might expect, most of the complaints came in when she had to turn people away who were not allowed to visit or when it was past visiting hours. Finally, I scheduled myself to sit at a visiting desk with the struggling employee, under the guise that I was evaluating overall procedures at the hospital visiting centers. It didn't take long for me to figure out her problem.

Just after 8PM, a man walked into the lobby, right past the "Visiting Hours Are Over" sign. The visiting center staff member beamed her famous smile toward him and said cheerfully, as she always did, "Good evening. Welcome to the hospital. How can we assist you?"

"I'm here to visit a friend", he replied. "He is a patient on the 7th floor."

To that the woman's huge and toothy grin seemed to even increase, and in the most pleasant and cheerful tone imaginable, she said, "Oh, I'm sorry, visiting hours ended at 8PM."

"I just drove 45 minutes to get here," he answered.

"I'm so sorry, Sir," she said brightly, "but the rules say visitation after 8PM is for immediate family only."

"Do you think this is funny?" he shot back at her. At that moment I knew exactly the nature of her problem. Her smile and cheerful nature was the only tool on her belt.

Having gone to scores of disturbance calls in hospitals over the years, I've observed many patterns of behavior that sparked or generated conflict and even violence. One of the things I've heard with great frequency from patients and visitors is, "What are you smiling at?" People have to be adaptable in their communication styles and know when to wear the appropriate expression.

Students of Vistelar's training programs are drilled to develop a *Showtime Mindset* that sets the tone for communication. Proper tone and volume of voice, as well as the appropriate expression are modeled, practiced, and reinforced. That's because it doesn't really matter what we say, if we don't say it well. The only way we can filter out our own moods and feelings is through practice and by raising the expectation for how staff interact with others. It's important that everyone in professional life understands the position of advantage is ours, and the onus for setting the tone for professional relationships is on us—not on our patients, clients, and customers.

If things aren't going well overall, then the fault partially lies in us. Ultimately, it is the fault of leaders for failing to prepare our staff through dedicated training. The stakes are high when we fail to train for what we do most as human service professionals, sales people, law enforcement officers, or anyone in a public job. And what we do most is communicate.

Joel Lashley

Chapter Four
The Basketball Coach
Universal Greeting

"The alternative to violence is dialogue."

Marshall McLuhan

It was a busier than usual Tuesday afternoon in the Emergency Department, and Dr. Jones was effectively running from one patient to the next. A fifteen-year-old girl named Megan presented with severe abdominal pain that morning, for which he had ordered several tests. Her latest test results were in, so he grabbed her chart and looked around hurriedly for her nurse, but she was nowhere in sight. Not having time to wait, he trotted over to the patient's room, slid the curtain open abruptly and stepped inside, while still skimming the chart.

When Dr. Jones finally looked up, he saw the patient lying in bed and a forty-something looking woman sitting in a chair next to her. The patient and her guest were smiling and it was obvious that he had interrupted a pleasant and lively conversation. He felt a sense of relief that he wasn't going to have to track down the parent to discuss his findings; and that both of them appeared to be in a good mood. The news he had wasn't life threatening but it wasn't pleasant either. With that in mind, Dr. Smith began his report.

"Hello again, Megan," he began. Megan simply stared at him with a look of anticipation on her face. Then he glanced over at her guest and introduced himself. "Hello, I'm Megan's Doctor. Her latest test results are back."

The woman smiled brightly up at him and said in a pleasant tone, "Hello. Pleased to meet you. Megan's been waiting patiently."

Again, Dr. Jones felt relieved, as she appeared to be a pleasant woman and he had already dealt with a couple angry mothers that day. "Well we have good news, and bad news," he continued. "Megan is not pregnant. However, she has two STDs, both of which are treatable. So it's not the end of the world."

The patient looked up at him with a familiar look of shock and fear on her face, so he just continued in an effort to calm her. "I have a social worker stopping in to talk to both of you about Megan being sexually active at such a young age. She will have advice on how to keep safe and answer any questions you might have. She will be able to offer counseling and help you figure out what to do next."

All in all it seemed like the encounter was going well, at least up to that point. However, there was one serious issue with that patient contact, ultimately resulting in a formal complaint, due to violations of hospital policy, HIPAA regulations, and both CMS and Joint Commission regulations and rules. The woman sitting next to Megan's bed was not her mother. She was, in fact, her basketball coach.

How could that situation have been avoided? One response might be to instruct healthcare providers to always introduce themselves, but would that have avoided this incident? Dr. Smith did, in fact, introduce himself. Perhaps the next step would be to instruct providers to always identify their patients, but hospitals are already doing that as well. They band each patient and instruct providers to check each patient's band to positively identify them. Still, patient ID bands don't prevent privacy issues with visitors. Maybe the situation could have been avoided if the physician had checked to see if the visitor had been wearing a parent pass. However, this particular hospital didn't issue passes of any kind. Then the answer must be to tell all providers to introduce themselves to everyone in the room at each and every patient contact. Problem solved! Really? Unfortunately, it's not that easy.

Speech is a psychomotor skill. You can't build psychomotor skills through a list of written instructions or policies. First you have to specify the skills required and then practice them. The skill that could have avoided this problem is the *Universal Greeting*. Simply stated, the *Universal Greeting* begins with a proper greeting, i.e., "Good morning", or "Good evening" followed by the providers name and department. "My name is Dr. Jones" followed by your reason for addressing someone, "I'm here to discuss your lab results." The next step is to ask a relevant question, which also gives the provider an opening to identify everyone in the room and determine who should be present or not.

Dr Jones:	"Good Afternoon, Megan. It's Dr. Jones. I stopped by to see how you're doing and show you your lab results."
Megan:	"Good, I guess."
Dr. Jones:	"Hello, Ma'am, I'm Doctor Jones, Megan's doctor."
Guest:	"Hello, Doctor."
Dr. Jones:	"I'm the physician on duty in the Emergency Department today. And you are?"
Guest:	"I'm Mrs. Brown."

Dr. Jones: "It's nice to meet you, Mrs. Brown. How do you know Megan?"

Guest: "I'm her basketball coach."

Although medicine is a very emotional and high stakes profession, it is very task driven. Every encounter is timed and the demands of the next waiting patient are forever on a providers mind. Medicine is physically and psychologically draining and the hours are long. It is also an information-driven profession and a provider's mind is always working at a fever pitch. The *Universal Greeting* would have avoided this very common but high stakes error. One that is committed everyday in hospitals all across America. The *Universal Greeting* has many benefits in all areas of medicine and preventing HIPPA violations is only one of them.

In healthcare, conflict is common. That conflict is often the result of poor initial contacts. One contact that is all too common is the *"who-the-hell-are-you"* contact. This statement is one that signals things are starting to go wrong and it's going to take a lot of effort to get back on the right track. The *Universal Greeting* can also eliminate this common pitfall in patient relations.

Like we stated earlier, nursing is a very task driven profession. One of those arduous yet routine and high-stakes tasks is patient triage. It is not uncommon for triage nurses to serve a long line of irritable patients and impatient visitors. That said, the one variable that an individual nurse has primary control of is how each encounter begins.

In many cases, patients are greeted by harried and stern nurses who are still recovering from uncomfortable and even frightening encounters with other challenging patients. Day in and day out, they experience arguments and threats from a small number of patients during the triage process. It can be so bad in some ERs and clinics, that nurses even draw straws to determine who gets stuck with triage.

Still, in most cases, nursing units seem to know who are their problem nurses. They are the nurses who constantly get in arguments during triage and send back patients for treatment in a bad mood. In my career, I've sat next to many triage nurses and observed how they worked. The ones that had all the problems had a few attributes in common.

Usually, they demonstrated poor eye contact, by staring down at their triage sheet and rarely making eye contact. Secondly, they usually presented an inappropriate expression. That is, they wore their hearts on their sleeves and their moods on their faces. If they were tired, angry, disgusted, or just plain hated to be the nurse stuck at triage, they wore those feelings on their faces. Finally, they treated their patients not as patients, but as the *next person in line*. In those cases, the encounter often went like this:

Nurse: "Next please."

Patient: "Yeah, I hurt my wrist at work."

Nurse: "Spell your first name."

Patient: "John Reed."

Nurse: "Just spell your first name, please."

Patient: "Look, my wrist really f***ing hurts!"

Nurse: "Just calm down, sir. We'll take care of your wrist."

Patient: "Don't tell me to f***ing calm down! My f***ing wrist is broken!"

Nurse: "Sir, please just calm down and spell your name!"

Patient: "Are you telling me you don't know how to f***ing spell John?!"

It seems obvious that the encounter could have gone better. You might also draw the conclusion that the man with the broken wrist was just a jerk or that he's just behaving that way because he is in pain. Both may have been true; nonetheless, the entire initial contact should have and could have gone much differently.

Nurse: "Good afternoon, my name is Lisa. I am the nurse that will check you in. What brings you to the hospital today?"

Patient: "Yeah, I hurt my wrist at work."

Nurse: "Oh my, I can see that. I'll check you in so we can take care of that arm as quickly as possible. Can you please take a seat right here?"

Patient: "It really hurts a lot."

Nurse: "Try not to move it. It may be best if we just cut your sleeve off."

Patient: "I don't care about the f***ing shirt, it hurts!"

Nurse: "I understand. We're going to manage your pain as quickly as we can. Just be aware there are families around. Try not to curse or frighten them, okay? I know it hurts."

Patient: "I'm sorry, I'm just upset."

Nurse: "Perfectly understandable, I would be too. Please take a seat so I can look at your wrist and take your vitals. Thank you. Now let's finish checking you in. How do you spell your first name?"

Patient: "My name is John"

Nurse: "Is John your full name, or Jonathon?"

Patient: "Jonathon."

Nurse: "Thank you. Now can you spell your last name?"

Patient: "Do you have to know all that right now?"

Nurse: "I have to find your records and register you, before we can order tests, see a doctor, or even prescribe medications. The sooner I check you in, the sooner we can see the doctor and get you out of pain."

Patient: "Okay, whatever. My name is Reed. That's R, E, E, D."

Nurse: "Thank you. What is your middle initial?"

By following the *Universal Greeting*, this nurse was able to set the tone for a better clinical relationship. Clinical relationships don't really start at the door. They start with the first time a patient sees a provider's face, hears their voice, and by the first words out of the provider's mouth. Despite what we might think, patients don't ultimately set the tone for a clinical relationship. Providers do that. It is the provider that is in a position of advantage when it comes to patient relationships, because providers are the ones wearing the scrubs, wearing the identification, and providing the skills necessary to treat a patient's illness or injury.

Professionals of any stripe only lose their professional advantage if they surrender it. The way they surrender it is usually by the words they use or don't use, and the styles in which they communicate. It's not as much the words we use, but our delivery style that makes the difference.

To be effective, providers must appear confident to their patients. That said, there is a huge gulf between arrogance and confidence, although it is easy to confuse these two very different states of mind. The *Universal Greeting* is the first step to establishing yourself as a confident and competent provider. Competent providers are happy to introduce themselves and state their business. Arrogant, indecisive, fearful, or incompetent providers are not. Even if the provider is highly competent, their communication style will determine their patients and peers perceptions.

That is why the *Universal Greeting* is inexorably tied to a provider's non-verbal communication. Again, it's all about perception. A provider's visual presence, signaled by their scrubs, identification cards, stethoscopes and other "badges of office", are the first element of the provider's presence. Worn, faded, unkempt clothing and poor hygiene are the obvious issues most providers already have well under control, but even the absence of an identification card can chip away at a provider's professional presence.

Hand washing is an important part of patient care and I think most everyone in healthcare gets that, now. But the hand washing ritual is not just an important part of infection control, but of professional presence as well. That's precisely why some hospitals and healthcare systems have wisely instructed their providers to wash their hands first and in the presence of their patients when they arrive in the room. It is a general rule that, if it doesn't happen in a patient's presence, it doesn't happen at all. Ironically, providers should assume their patients don't assume anything! So, something as simple as washing your hands in front of them goes a long way to earning a patient's trust and confidence. Whenever providers are in the presence of their patients they are on stage. Things as simple as taking the time to sit when you talk with patients or showing them their x-rays and explaining them, are all part of a provider's stage presence.

Wearing the appropriate expression or showing your *on-stage face (Showtime Mindset)*; and using a supportive and confident tone and volume of voice are all part of effective communication. Combined with a *Universal Greeting*, these things are how we begin to establish more therapeutic relationships. It is also how we avoid relationships that are compatible with uncooperative and ultimately violent behavior.

Have you ever seen a fight in a church? How about a bank? Probably not. Have you ever seen a fight in school? How about at a bar? If you went to school as a kid or spent much time in local taverns, you probably have seen a fight. At the outset, the answers seem obvious. Kids fight and so do drunks. But is that all there is to it?

If you've ever worked in a hospital, you possibly have seen a fight. I've spent years in hospitals and I've seen scores of them. Why? Is it just because the stakes are so high in hospitals? Certainly illness and issues revolving around life and death contribute to the level of conflict in hospitals. That said, perhaps there is more to the story.

Do you think people fight a lot in libraries? It seems like a silly question, and the answer appears to be obvious. In fact, fights are unusual in libraries. I've spent hundreds of hours in libraries and I've never seen one. Why not? Is it simply because the stakes are lower than in a hospital? After all, it's just a library. Or is it because only peace loving people read books? Let's examine that premise. What kinds of people go to the libraries these days?

Libraries are much different places than when I was a kid. I used to ride my bike to the library along with a lot of other kids. In those days, the only things there were books and magazines. One of the things that make them so different now is computers. In any given library, there are several computers. Even in small branch libraries in large cities, there are typically rows of computers.

These days, many libraries are only about half stocked with books. Instead, their shelves are stocked with DVDs and CDs offering hundreds of movies and musical recordings. Along with all that media are new clientele who previously would never have set foot in a library. But also there are all those computers and WiFi connections for laptops.

What exactly are all those people doing on those computers? Perhaps doing homework or searching for employment? No doubt a few are using them for sensible purposes. A lot of them are accessing social media and email. A significant portion of them are accessing or trying to access pornography. In some libraries, pornography and its overt exposure to other patrons — even children — have become unbearable. The public library in many cities has also become a default homeless shelter. But given all these challenges, fights are still relatively rare in libraries. Why? The answer lies in the *Social Contract* of the library.

What happens if you talk above a whisper in most libraries? What happens if your cell phone starts ringing in your pocket? The first thing that happens is that everyone around you turns and looks at you disapprovingly. You experience the disapproval of *the herd*.

So what would happen if you continued to talk loudly despite everyone looking at you disapprovingly? The librarian would likely approach you and ask you to be quiet. That's the next layer of the *Social Contract*, the intervention of *the leader*.

By then, most people would get with the program. But what if you told the librarian to mind her own business? Would she just go away? In all likelihood, she would ask you to leave. And if you refused she would call the police — *the enforcer*. When the police arrived, if you refused to leave when they asked, they would arrest you — *the consequence*. In essence, you got arrested because you were loud at the library!

The reason arguments and fights are rare in libraries is because many of the gateway behaviors that lead to arguments and fights are loud and violate the *Social Contract* of libraries. Silence in libraries is an expectation of behavior that is universally understood. Indirectly, the expectation of behavior in a library works to create an iron clad *Social Contract* that is incompatible with violence. That is, a social contract that is set, supported and sustained by four elements: *the herd, the leader, the enforcer,* and *the consequence*.

You see, the big mean angry biker from chapter one knows exactly how to behave in church. If he goes to church, whether just for family functions, for holidays, or regularly, he sits when told to sit, stands when told to stand, sings when told to sing, passes the collection plate, and greets his neighbor when prompted by the pastor. This is the very same person who probably manages all his relationships, both personal and professional, through intimidation.

When he walks into a bank, angry about his paycheck being short and the bills piling up, he simply gets in line and quietly walks through a maze, waiting his turn to see a teller. There is not a whole lot of active reinforcement for the *Social Contract* of a bank, but everyone knows what will happen if you start yelling and cursing. The police are sure to be called and your account will likely be closed.

So why do so many people go to hospitals and start yelling, cursing, and even threatening? Is it because people aren't sure how to behave? Are hospitals and clinics themselves partly responsible for all that bad behavior? What is wrong with the social contract of healthcare and why is it seemingly so compatible with anti-social behavior and ultimately violence? If the elements of an enforceable *Social Contract* are: *the herd, the leader, the enforcer,* and *the consequence,* what parts are missing from healthcare? The best way to illustrate that is through another story. A story I've used many times in training.

On one occasion I was called to conduct a risk assessment on the father of an infant admitted to the NICU. He had reportedly made several threats toward staff on the unit. They were described as implied or "veiled" threats. While investigating the complaint, I attempted to interview as many involved staff as possible.

One nurse said that the father was "grumpy", always glaring at the nurses and seeming to stand guard outside his baby's room. He would just stand there, with his arms folded and scowl at passersby. He rarely spoke, but when he did, he was always brief and "intense" as she put it. Once as she walked by he asked her, "Who is that guy?"

She said, "That's the charge nurse? Do you need to talk to him?"

"No, just tell him to stay the hell out of my baby's room," he replied threateningly.

I asked her what she did and she said she did nothing. She also didn't report it or even record it. I asked her if she told the charge nurse. She said yes, but they both laughed it off. I asked the charge nurse myself about it and he said, not surprisingly, that such remarks from parents are, "part of the job."

Another nurse I interviewed had a lot to say about the grumpy father. She complained that he was always there and always keeping vigil, as described by the other nurse. She said he asked her once for a doctor's name, while pointing her out at the nurses' station. Thinking it odd, she asked him why he wanted to know her name. She said he answered, "So I know who to shoot if my baby dies." Almost surprisingly, she didn't report that to the doctor in question. She did discuss it with her fellow nurses who decided that it was a hollow threat and, you guessed it, "part of the job."

Finally, a young nurse noticed the grumpy father standing vigil outside his baby's room and asked him if she could get him anything, perhaps some coffee or some juice. She said he replied, "How about a gun?" After that final remark, the nursing supervisor on duty decided to call security.

My background investigation hadn't revealed a criminal record, so after my investigation it was time for me to address the grumpy father. I requested a back-up officer to assist me for safety reasons and when I voiced my intention to some of the nursing and medical staff on the unit, they objected. They worried that confronting him would just make him angry. After some discussion to reassure them, I approached the patient's father.

While he was standing guard at his son's door, I approached him wearing a friendly smile. At 10 feet away, he noticed me approaching. We made eye contact and he watched me cautiously as I drew closer.

At about five feet away, well outside of arms length, I began my initial contact.

"Hello Mr. Smith. My name is Joel and I work for hospital security. I heard you were upset today and I wanted to stop by and see if I could help. How is your baby doing today?" I asked about his baby in an attempt to focus his attention toward his baby and away from the stress and anger he might be feeling. This is a form of distraction that will often keep people centered on what's most important. We can use this method of distraction, during our *Universal Greeting*, as the relevant question to begin non-escalation. Questions like, "How are you feeling today?" or "How is your wife, is she resting better?" will often refocus someone's attention away from their anger and stress. It also is an important method of showing empathy.

"He is doing okay," he replied, maintaining his cautious expression.

"That's great!" I said smiling. "Are you going to get to take him home soon?"

"We don't know for sure, yet." he replied. "But they may be moving him to another floor soon."

"Well that sounds encouraging. If he's leaving the NICU, then he must be getting better," I said cheerfully.

"I guess so," he replied for the first time smiling a little.

We continued with a little small talk and I asked him how his wife was holding up, as I could see her in the room attending to her baby. After that, I broached the subject for which I was making the contact. "So I understand that you've been a little tense, while your son's been with us. The reason I am here is because of some concerns about some comments you've made."

"I'm just sticking up for my baby!" he said now getting a little agitated, but not shouting or being inappropriate.

"I understand, that's our job as parents, right?" I asked.

"Yes, that's right. I also want to teach him to stand up for himself," he replied.

With that, I stretched out my arm and pointed down the hall towards a conference room. "I respect that, Mr. Smith. Why don't we take a seat over here and discuss what's bothering you."

"We can talk right here," he replied.

"We could do that, but I don't want anyone else hearing your business. We can talk privately over there," I replied.

After a moment's deliberation, he shrugged and said, "Fine. I don't know what this is all about, but we can talk."

When we arrived at the conference room, I motioned for him to enter first. My back up officer had been instructed to remain outside of the room, but in earshot. Staying close behind, I pointed to a chair at the other side of the table for Mr. Smith to take a seat, saying simply, "Take a seat over there, please. We can talk privately in here."

Previously, I had removed all chairs but two from the room. I placed one chair in the corner of the room and left the empty space at the table, nearest the door. That gave me the opportunity to retrieve the cornered chair and place it closest to the door for myself, so I was between him and my exit. That way, if things got out of control, I could easily escape. I then closed the door, but left it cracked. This gives the subject the feeling that we aren't totally alone. It also gives him the feeling that that he is not isolated or trapped. This is a common safety routine that I teach my students. After setting the stage, I continued my initial contact with Mr. Smith.

"Thank you for joining me in here, Mr. Smith. Like I said, I wanted to talk to you about some comments you reportedly made to some of our staff on the unit." He remained silent so I continued, "It's been reported that you made some threats. Can you tell me what has you so upset and why you might threaten our staff?"

"I didn't threaten anyone," he said sheepishly.

"Did you ask what a doctor's name was and said that you wanted to know who to shoot if your baby dies?" I said calmly with a look of concern.

"I didn't mean any of that. I'm just sticking up for my family!" he said tersely.

"I appreciate that, but you can't threaten to shoot people. You understand that, right?"

"Yeah, I know, but I didn't mean it. It's a free country and I can say what I want," he said defiantly.

"Well. Mr. Smith, you can't threaten to hurt people. And it's been reported to me that you've threatened to hurt people a couple of times, are intimidating to the staff, and even asked one of them for a gun. You may have been trying to be sarcastic, Mr. Smith, but you are scaring people and we can't have that," I said.

As the discussion continued, we discussed his concerns. The interesting thing was that he didn't have any specific complaints about his baby's treatment or the staff. He was very young, under stress, obviously, and didn't appear to have very good coping skills. He advised me that he and his wife had no family support. I explained that he had the right to complain to nursing supervisors and seek assistance if needed from hospital counselors, chaplains, and patient relations staff. I also set limits on any future behaviors, stating that if any more threats were made he could lose the right to visit his own baby in the hospital. This of course shocked him.

"You can't stop me from visiting my own baby!" he replied.

"Sir, that's not what we want. But if you threaten our staff, the police become involved. Your wife and baby need you here with them. So if you have problems, I'm showing you the right way to handle them so you don't get in trouble and lose your visitation rights."

After our discussion, he assured me that there would be no more threats. Also, his baby's health was progressing nicely, eliminating any apparent motive for violence. Based on his apologetic tone and demeanor, I was satisfied that his threats weren't genuine. That said, I filed a safety plan for nursing staff, which included a zero-tolerance for threatening or intimidating behavior, requiring an immediate security response. I then completed a routine security risk assessment for the medical record.

He asked to speak to a counselor, so I put in a social work referral. I reassured him that we had no intentions of pressing any charges; based on the information we had at that time. A routine police report was made, so I advised him that a police detective, as a matter of routine, might question him.

When we stood to leave the room, the grumpy father stretched out his hand and offered it for me to shake, "Thanks for not throwing me out. I'm really sorry for all this. Please tell everyone I'm not that kind of guy." I shook Mr. Smith's hand and wished him well.

The Smith family had been moved to another unit while their baby recovered and within a few days their baby was discharged. While they were there, I checked in with the nursing staff, all who had nothing but good to say about the Smiths. I even popped in on Mr. Smith to ask how things were going. I even got to where I looked forward to our brief meetings and I like to think he did as well. A couple days after their discharge, the nursing unit received a card from the Smith's. They also sent one to the NICU where all the threats had originated. In the cards they heaped praise on the staff, thanking them for their care.

Chapter Five
The Cold Supper Tray
Beyond Active Listening

"There is, however, a limit at which forbearance ceases to be a virtue."
Edmund Burke

One evening, while supervising security in a hospital, I was sent to a nursing unit subsequent to an assault on a nurse. The security team arrived ahead of me and the situation had already quieted down. The officers and I debriefed the incident among ourselves, before they returned to regular duties. They reported to me that the floor was already quiet when they arrived so I stayed behind to tie up the loose ends. No injuries were reported and all appeared well; however, when I debriefed the nursing staff a different story started to unfold.

The nursing supervisor complained that this particular mother of a patient was verbally abusive and sometimes even threatening towards nursing staff. I asked how long this had been going on and she said about a week. When I asked if she'd reported anything to security before tonight she said she hadn't nor had anyone else. When

I looked through the medical record there were no social work or nursing notations about the mother's supposed weeklong abusive behavior. It was unfortunate that the unit staff had waited so long to ask for help. In all likelihood, this incident could have been avoided if we had been able to rein in this mother's behavior when it first started. Addressing her behavior at this late stage was going to be much more difficult.

The incident went something like this: the patient's evening meal had been delivered, along with a visitor's meal for the mother. The mother was displeased with the meal and threw her tray at the patient's nurse. The tray missed her, but smashed against the wall causing the nurse to run from the room. After hearing this, I decided to speak to the mother.

"Don't go in there!" said the nursing supervisor. "You'll just make things worse."

"Her behavior was pretty outrageous," I replied. "You also said she's been going on like this for a while. Don't you think we need to get to the bottom of things and set some limits on her behavior?" I asked.

"Not right now. We just got her calmed down!" she pleaded.

"I understand how you feel, but I have to make an assessment and set some limits," I replied. "I'll try not to make things any worse."

When I arrived at the room the door was half open. It was dark inside and quiet, except for the low volume of the television set. I knocked on the doorframe and the mother said, "What do you want?" in a stern tone of voice. With that I opened the door all the way and stood just inside the doorframe, where I could see the room and assess for any hidden dangers. I could also exit the situation quickly if she decided to start throwing things again! When I saw the scene was safe, I started in with my *Universal Greeting*.

"Hello, Ma'am. My name is Joel. I'm the security supervisor on duty." She just stared at me blankly, so I continued. "The reason I'm here is because of the incident that just happened. I need to get your side of things. Can you tell me what has you upset tonight?"

"I'm not upset, everything is fine, I don't need to talk to you," she said, matter-of-factly.

"I understand what you're saying ma'am, but I have to talk to you about the incident. Can you please tell me what happened?" While talking, I had entered the room and closed the space between us to about five feet.

Then she looked up at me and continued, "These nurses are disrespectful. They're rude and act like they're better than me. And they aren't taking care of my child properly!"

"Well, I understand now why you're angry. Have you complained to the charge nurse or a supervisor?" Before she could answer, I blurted, "How's your daughter doing, by the way?" This is an important point in the conversation for healthcare workers. Again, in healthcare we have a built in *emotional or practical appeal.* Drawing a patient's attention to their own condition, or even a visitor's or family member's attention to their loved one's condition, can go a long way to showing *Empathy* and resetting their state of mind.

"She's doing better," replied the mother.

"Great, is she going home soon?" I asked.

"We were supposed to go home tomorrow," she answered in a trembling voice.

"Well, I hope she is well enough to go home soon, if not tomorrow." I then continued with some probing questions to clarify the situation in my mind. "Can you tell me what happened tonight? The nurses said you threw a tray."

"My food tray was cold! I'm tired of being treated like this!" she said tersely.

"Let me see if I understand what you're saying," I asked. At this point, I was preparing to *Paraphrase* what she had just said. Paraphrasing is a powerful tool in conversation. It's a way of getting people to focus, as everyone generally will give you their full attention whenever you say you are going to tell them your thoughts on what they've just said. You can even politely interrupt by saying something like "let me tell you what I think you mean."

Paraphrasing also serves as a sort of mirror that reflects the other person's behavior back at them. "So you're saying that you threw your tray at the nurse, smashing glasses and plates on the wall and causing her to run from the room because your dinner was cold? I have to write a report so I really want to make sure I get your side of things." At that point she hung her head and started to sob quietly, so I just continued. "Ma'am, I know something's wrong and I want to help. I don't think you threw your tray at that nurse just because your meal was cold. Can you tell me what's really wrong so I can help you?"

"Yeah, well," she said softly before continuing. "My no good husband gambled our rent money. My daughter is getting out tomorrow and we don't have anywhere to go."

That was my opening to *Summarize* the situation for her and move towards some resolution. "I'm glad you confided in me, Ma'am. Here's what I can do. With your permission, I can ask the on-duty hospital social worker to stop up tonight. She may have some options to help in this situation. We don't want to discharge your daughter to the street. Your doctor and the hospital administration will want to know what's going on and will try to help if you let them. Also, if you want to see about counseling for your husband's gambling, she will have resources for him."

She sighed deeply before answering in a sheepish tone, "Yes, I would like to talk to someone."

"I'm only too glad to help you and your daughter. However, you understand that if you had hit that nurse with that tray, you'd probably have been arrested for an assault. Then you would be in jail, your daughter would still be in here, and your rent would still be unpaid."

"I'm sorry. I wasn't trying to hit her," she replied.

"I'm really glad you didn't. If at any time you feel that you're being treated unfairly, talk to the charge nurse or a supervisor. You could also ask to talk to someone from patient relations. Now that you know what to do if there are problems, I'm asking you to please stop yelling and cursing at your daughter's nurses. I can't help you unless you show them respect." She nodded in agreement, so I continued, "There are also other kids on this floor and this has to be a safe, quiet, and appropriate environment for them as well as your daughter."

Before leaving the unit, I debriefed the nursing staff. I shared with them her assurances that she would show them respect. I asked that they address cursing, yelling, and name calling immediately and that they should call security for support, before things got out of hand again. Perhaps, most importantly, I shared the mother's perspective that she felt disrespected by some of the nurses. I also shared that she was struggling with some very profound family issues, causing her to be fearful about her daughter's future after discharge.

The patient and her mother were on the unit for another three days without incident. I checked in often to see how things were going and the nurses related that the mother had "opened up" to many of them and was generally pleasant. The mother related to me that the nursing staff was much more supportive and approachable. On the final day the nursing supervisor asked me what many doctors, nurses, social workers, and hospital security people have asked me over the years, after dealing with difficult patients and families. She asked, "What exactly did you say to her?"

In the final analysis, it isn't as much as what we say with our words as what we "do" with them. As for the angry mother in the preceding story, I established communication with a *Universal Greeting* and empathized with her situation, while not entirely agreeing with her point of view. We can show *Empathy* with someone's situation without legitimizing bad behavior, by simply acknowledging their illness, their situation, or even their anger. I also asked questions to *Clarify* her point of view, while mining for details. People aren't usually forthcoming when being called-out on their behavior, so clarifying questions are essential for getting them to open up. Then, I shared my understanding of both the situation and her point of view by *Paraphrasing*. By doing so I was able to focus her attention and reflect her behavior back for her to examine objectively. Finally, I was able to *Summarize*—problem solve, set limits on future bad behaviors and offer appropriate solutions for future problems.

These techniques are part of the skill set of the *Beyond Active Listening* tactic that providers are trained to use in Vistelar's conflict management training course. By building competence in this tactic and applying it early in the cycle of violence, situations like the one above can be avoided and clinical relationships can be strengthened even under the most trying circumstances. Going *Beyond Active Listening* isn't just for setting limits on known behaviors, but also for getting to the root of both real and potential problems.

Every provider knows patients who had poor outcomes and were still grateful for the care they received. They also know patients who had stellar outcomes but still filed several complaints and treated staff disrespectfully despite every effort being made to ensure their satisfaction. A patient's perception of the care they received is connected not only to the outcomes of therapy, but also to the environment in which that therapy was delivered. Was it quiet? Was it safe? Was it clean? Was the staff friendly and approachable? Any one of these lynch pins, if pulled out of place, can collapse the overall favorable perception of the quality of care.

This may be especially true, in relation to the *Gateway Behaviors of Violence*. If a patient's life is on the line, their choice of hospital is primarily based on its resources and reputation, within the constraints of their financial resources and insurance policy. But for routine hospitalizations and urgent care needs, they will more likely choose comfort and safety over reputation and even location. This is a dynamic I've witnessed many times from both sides. I have worked in top-notch facilities that people refused to patronize because the perception was that they were unsafe. I've also worked in others that were out of the way and of average reputation that people drove long distances to get to because the perception was that they were safer than the ones in their own community. Sometimes that perception was connected to a hospital or clinics' location in a high-crime area or just the fact that it was located in a major city. Often, however, it was connected to something they had seen or heard when they were once in the emergency room at that hospital or visiting one of its clinics. Sometimes, it was based solely on its reputation as an unsafe place.

The *Universal Greeting* combined with *Beyond Active Listening* form a skill set providers can use to set and maintain a *Social Contract* that promotes patient satisfaction. That said, the pendulum swings both ways. One of the things providers complain about a lot is the tension that some patients and even family members bring to the bedside. Often, that tension is something they can't put their finger on. Sometimes it's just a look, a sigh, or just a "feeling" that patients and visitors bring to a therapeutic relationship. "What's the harm?" you might ask. The harm caused by undefined "tension" is that it directly impacts the perception of the care the patient is receiving.

Complaints are more likely generated based on a patient's or family member's attitude and have little or nothing to do with the actual quality of care that they received. The point being that patient satisfaction isn't solely connected to the quality of care, but also to the beliefs and attitudes the patient brings to the environment of care. But what, if anything, can we do about that?

People can be categorized into three personality types for the purpose of training. The first are "yes" people. They are the ones who are positive in their dealings with everyone. "Yes" people are the ones who are generous and understanding even when things don't always go well. However, if "Yes" people are handled improperly, even their goodwill can be eroded.

Then there are "No" people, who are hard to satisfy and overly suspicious. They are the ones who often refuse to cooperate, the first time they are asked to do something. However, in the hands of a skillful communicator, they can be persuaded to comply.

The last are "passive-aggressive" people. They appear to be "yes" people, but are actually "no" people." Passive-aggressive people hide their real purpose, their real feelings, and their real attitudes. Their complaints come out of left field and they only make them if there is no personal risk involved. These can be the toughest people to manage. Passive-aggressive patients may appear satisfied and never complain to the provider face-to-face, but then throw them under the bus to other providers, administrators, other patients and visitors.

Passive-aggressive staff members can do serious damage to the environment of care. Passive-aggressive behavior is a category of conflict on which I am frequently asked for advice, whether it's peer-to-peer or directed against providers from patients and families. Among peers, in the healthcare profession, it is commonly referred to as *lateral violence* or *systemic bullying*. According to the American Nurses Association, well over half of the nurses they surveyed in 2001 reported having been verbally abused or threatened by peers or people in authority.

A 2004 study from the Institute for Safe Medication Practices found that 48 percent of nurses, pharmacists and other healthcare professionals reported experiencing verbal abuse from peers and 43 percent reported intimidating and threatening body language. Perhaps most disturbing is that 40 percent of respondents reported "keeping quiet" when noticing medication errors due to an intimidating colleague, yet another way that violence affects patient health and safety.

Lateral violence from peers, just like violence experienced from patients and families, also affects staff performance by its negative impact on overall morale and increasing absenteeism and turnover. This is a particular concern considering we are currently experiencing a national nursing shortage. Therefore, lateral violence, just like any other form of healthcare violence, is affecting the public health. Studies have also documented the negative effect of lateral violence on patient health and safety, while still others have revealed its impact on providers themselves. The effects of lateral violence in healthcare include higher levels of anxiety and anger that can lead to depression, hypertension, and even coronary heart disease.

Recommendations for dealing with lateral violence range from raising awareness to policies protecting whistle blowers and zero-tolerance for bullying. But how do we manage behaviors, such as gossiping, ostracism, excluding and the withholding of information? What about intimidating behavior, such as the looks, sighs, and "feeling" that can permeate an office or nursing unit? *Beyond Active Listening* is clearly one skill set we can teach clinicians and managers to protect their working environments and empower providers to protect themselves. Especially since nursing is thought to be one of the professions where lateral violence is most prevalent and its affects most devastating. Bullying is no secret among members of the healthcare profession and perhaps that's why the expression, "Nurses eat their young" is so widely known.

What about those patients and family members who negatively impact the environment of care and ultimately affect their own outcomes? When patients and visitors are rolling their eyes, addressing us in an irritated tone of voice, or conspicuously ignoring us, we need to call those behaviors out into the sunlight. Skilled providers using the *Beyond Active Listening* technique can set and maintain a better, safer, and more therapeutic *Social Contract* with their patients.

"Hello, Mrs. Davis. I'm Julia, your mother's nurse this evening," she said smiling and in whispered tones, as her patient was sleeping. "I just stopped in to get her vitals. Can I get you anything afterwards?"

"No," replied Mrs. Davis shortly, never looking up from her magazine to make eye contact.

"Her pulse is strong and her blood pressure is very stable tonight, that's good," whispered the pleasant nurse.

"Whatever you say," said the visitor, while rolling her eyes, shaking her head and smirking disapprovingly.

"Ma'am, I know you've been here a long time and you seem worried. Can I help? Maybe I can answer some questions?"

"There's nothing you can say to me," said the visitor.

"Well I can see that you're upset about something and I just want to help."

"I'm not upset," replied the visitor.

"Okay. I just want you to know that I'm here for you if you need anything or if you have any concerns. It's no fun being cooped up all day and worrying about your mother. Can I get you some blankets, pillows, some coffee or something? Maybe I could check around and find some better magazines?" she offered while wearing a look somewhere between a smile and a look of concern.

The visitors grim face softened and she looked the nurse in the eye for the first time, saying, "I'm sorry I'm such a b***h."

"Oh, not at all, Mrs. Davis," replied the nurse.

"I don't mean to take it out on you. You're such a sweet girl. My mom is lucky you're here for her. I'm just tired and worried, like you said. And these magazines do suck," she said, laughing.

"Yeah, I bet they do. Everyone takes the good ones home. Let me see what else is around to read."

That was an example of a real encounter between a nurse and a visitor—a visitor who had been reported many times as being a hard case. Usually, nurses just kept quiet when she was in the room, not addressing her at all. Some of them even wore stern expressions, while getting in and out fast, spending as little time as possible with the patient. Others, tried to kill her with kindness, but just ended up being laughed at or dismissed.

What made this nurses' encounter different was that she began with a *Universal Greeting*. Then she *Empathized* with the woman's situation. Then she asked questions to *Clarify* if there was anything wrong or if she had an unmet need. Then she performed a modified *Paraphrase*, even though she didn't have much to work with, by stating, "I can see you're upset about something." Finally she *Summarized* by saying, "I just want you to know I'm here for you, if you need anything." By going *Beyond Active Listening*, we can get to the real meaning of what people are saying. We can also open an opportunity to set limits on unsafe or anti-therapeutic behaviors. Most of all, we can begin to set a *Social Contract* that is compatible with healthy outcomes and incompatible with violent ones.

Joel Lashley

Chapter Six
"I Know You Are Upset, But..."
Redirections, Persuasion Sequence

"Don't raise your voice, improve your argument."
Bishop Desmond Tutu

I was engaged in a heated exchange with a man who was denied visitation by the patient herself, his own wife. She had made clear her wish not to see him and asked that he not be allowed up to her room. His expressions ran up and down the scale from disgust, to disbelief, to anger. Outwardly, he shot up and down the emotional scale from crying to threatening.

"This is really stupid! You can't stop me from seeing my own wife!" he lamented.

"I appreciate that you feel that way, Sir, but I'm not stopping you from seeing her, she is. She doesn't want to see you right now," I replied.

"Can you just let me talk to her on the phone?" he pleaded.

"I wish I could, but she refused to take any calls from you,"

I answered.

The exchange went on that way for minutes, with him pleading and providing excuses; and me just acknowledging his objections and redirecting his thoughts to logical conclusions.

"I'll just go up there anyway, you can't stop me!" he threatened.

"I understand you're angry, but that will just make things worse for you. I can't just let you run up the elevator and start fighting with your wife. Do you think she will be less angry with you if you cause a scene? Will you cooperate with me or do I need to just call for back up?"

At that the man looked me straight in the eye and blurted, "Yeah well, you're fat!"

I just looked down at the potbelly that was straining the buttons of my shirt and smiled. Then I looked up at him and simply said, "Really? I'm glad you said something. Maybe we caught it in time. I better get a gym membership."

Then the man just shook his head and chuckled, saying, "Okay, okay, you win. I'll talk to her later when she's not being such a b***h."

Communication breakdowns lead to conflict and violence. An engaged response is a give-and-take process that leads to resolution. An active verbal engagement may be infused verbal resistance. Even if you're in control of your own emotions and engaged in problem solving, your patient may not be there yet. Cursing, disagreement, challenges and disrespectful comments may be directed at you. Illogical explanations or solutions may be offered. Questions may be prompted by emotion or by someone just trying to be difficult. Excuses may be offered or even implied threats. All of these very natural distractions tend to derail communication and generate verbal resistance. The goal is to excise the emotion.

We are all human and certain things just make us angry. Motivated difficult people will find your weak spots or *"Conflict Triggers"* and exploit them in an effort to knock you off balance and take control of the clinical relationship. In the medical profession, all of us are just trying to provide the best treatment and environment of care for patients. When all you are trying to do is help, why is it that you sometimes encounter resistance? Police officers face this dilemma too. All professionals face this challenge. The strategy is to build *Triggers Guard* over your *Conflict Triggers* so they can't be so easily exploited. By recognizing your triggers ahead of time, by identifying what offends you, infuriates you, or just plain drives you crazy, you can be ready for them when they pop up.

The best way to handle these *Conflict Triggers* is to use the *Rediretions* tactic. The "I know you are upset, but can you work with me?" approach is the formula for diffusing and disempowering any emotional assault. *Rediretions* come in many forms like the humorous example above. But they also come in the form of pre-planned, practiced responses like the examples below:

- I understand...

- I appreciate your concern...

- I would feel the same way...

- I can see that you are really frustrated...

Statements that begin in this way intercept negative comments and acknowledge them in a positive way. As any boxer or martial artist knows, deflecting a strike not only protects from injury, it also provides a positive opportunity. Acknowledging a person's comment is especially powerful if used in combination with *Empathy*.

- I see that you are upset and I appreciate your concern...

- I know this must be difficult for you and I can hear that you're worried...

The *Rediretions* tactic is given context when the acknowledgement is immediately followed up by redirective language. The words "but" or "however" help to transition to solution-oriented language and help focus on problem solving rather than problem creating. Below are some examples of what we're talking about.

- I know you are upset, but…
- I can see your concern, however…
- I know you are frustrated and maybe I would feel the same way, nonetheless…

The solutions then offered might be as simple as…

- …could you please work with me?
- …would you help me help you?
- …we need to wait and see what the doctor thinks.

Putting this all together, *Redirections* end up sounding like this:

- I can see that you are upset but we need to wait until the test results come back and that can unfortunately take up to an hour. Can you work with me here?
- I know this must be difficult and I would probably be upset too under these circumstances. However, if you will work with me we can make sure that your child gets the exact care he needs.

Redirections are a way of inserting a tactical pause in a situation before our emotions over-ride our intellect. Childlike tantrum behaviors are only fed by childlike behavior in return. Our adult response, with the proper tone that is not authoritarian but caring, coupled with our calm response and demeanor, can re-assure the most emotionally out-of-control person that we are in control and can help.

I was sent to the nursing unit one night because a family court in another jurisdiction had requested that our hospital take temporary physical custody of an infant who was being treated for suspicious injuries. The baby had been flown to us by medevac helicopter from a neighboring state. The state had also faxed over the court order taking custody of the child. After meeting with the hospital manager on duty and the unit supervisor, the task fell on me to inform the baby's mother. I called the Child Protective Services agent involved in the case, to get specific instructions and prepare for the conversation ahead of me. It would turn out to be one of the most difficult conversations of my career.

When I arrived at the room it was dark, as only the light above the vanity was on and glowing dimly through the narrow window on the door. I knocked, but there was no answer. Slowly cracking the door, I could hear the mother weeping softly somewhere in a dark corner of the room. The nursing staff said she was alone, so I opened the door a little wider, stood in the doorway, and began with a *Universal Greeting*.

"Hello Ma'am, my name is Joel Lashley, I'm the Supervising Security Officer on duty in the hospital tonight. The reason I'm here is to inform you of where we are in the investigation concerning your baby's injuries." She started to sob openly now, so I took a deep breath and continued. I tried my usual practical appeal, by looking over at the crib and asking, "How is your baby resting now?" She didn't answer but only continued to sob deeply.

"I know this is very difficult, but I have to explain what's happening. Your state has taken temporary custody of your child and placed him in our physical custody until our doctors can complete their evaluation of your baby's injuries. Until then, you will not be able to visit. You have a court date on Monday that I need to tell you about and I have some paperwork to give you." The young mom began to cry openly now, so I just continued slowly and gently. "Your baby is safe here with us. He will get all that he needs and you can call whenever you like to get updates on him. If you have any questions for the nurses before you go, they will be happy to answer them. No decision about your child's future custody has been made yet. You just need to cooperate for the time being, as these things take a little time."

Just then, a fierce looking woman, who turned out to be the grandmother, pushed passed me and into the room. She went directly to the crib and picked up the sleeping baby, causing his IV lines and monitoring wires to dangle from his limbs in a tangled mess. "Ma'am, please put the baby down. He's injured and you don't want to make things worse," I said.

"No one is taking my grandchild from us!" she shouted as the baby began to cry.

"No one wants to take your baby, Ma'am, but he has to stay with us until things get cleared up…"

Interrupting me, she blurted, "We're leaving!"

"Ma'am, we have a couple good options here. You can put the baby down and, with the mother's permission, I can answer any questions you have. But, if you insist on trying to leave with that baby, I'll have to stop you. If you struggle and injure the baby, you'll be arrested."

"I don't care!" she shouted.

"Also, I have to file a report on how things go tonight. I want to write that you were concerned about your grandchild's health, asked a lot of questions, and cooperated with us. I don't want to write that you fought with us and manhandled the injured baby. What do you want me to write, Ma'am? It's all up to you."

After a few seconds of processing what I just said, the grandmother started to gently place the baby back in its crib. "I don't know who you think you are," she said, while still cooperating. "Do you feel like a big man taking people's babies away?" Just then the baby's father and grandfather walked in the room. The grandfather started in by saying, "What the hell is going on here?"

At that moment, the baby's mother said her first words, "Stop! All of you stop and leave him alone! He's the only person, since all this happened who hasn't treated me like a criminal!" Ultimately, the family cooperated and did just as I had hoped for them. They asked a lot of questions, showed their concern and love for their baby, and cooperated with the terms of the court order. Before leaving, the father and grandfather thanked me and shook my hand. The mother even gave me a hug.

The story above was an example of Vistelar's *Persuasion Sequence* in action. First, by beginning with a *Universal Greeting*, I was able to establish communication with a young mother in distress. Then when resistance was encountered I was able to manage the contact, by use of the *Persuasion Sequence*. First, by asking the grandmother to comply by putting the baby down and then by setting context for her, in other words, telling her why it was in her best interest to cooperate. Finally, I was able to generate voluntary cooperation by presenting the options; thereby, helping her to understand her choices, both good and bad. The options stage is in a very real sense, a reality check. In the majority of cases, even when under stress, most people will take the best option offered to them.

The genius of the *Persuasion Sequence* is that it causes both the provider and the patient to think clearly under pressure. That's because speech is a psychomotor skill, just like a golf swing. Through proper modeling, followed by practice and repetition, muscle memory is achieved. Once ingrained, the *Persuasion Sequence* provides a cognitive template, by which both patient and clinician can think clearly even when angry, frightened, or confused. The clinician is guided by their training and the patient is guided by the professional presence and voice of the provider. It's as simple as that.

Through proper modeling, training and practice, healthcare professionals can become proficient crisis communicators. In the majority of cases, a well-done *Persuasion Sequence* is effective even in seemingly impossible situations. Later in my career, I succeeded so often using the *Persuasion Sequence* that I was actually surprised when people didn't cooperate. At the beginning of my career, especially before training in Vistelar's conflict management methodologies, I was more often surprised when they did cooperate!

That may have been partially a function of experience; however, I've known many police officers, physicians, and supervisors who struggled their entire career, by never getting much cooperation from the people they served. In my own case, I believe my poor communication skills early in my career were a function of four dynamics: 1) A lack of experience. 2) A misunderstanding of my role, believing that my job was simply to enforce the rules. 3) The ingrained belief in healthcare that patient or family centered care is incompatible with setting limits on bad behavior and enforcing polices — even the law. 4) Training based solely on de-escalation theory instead of including non-escalation and Crisis Intervention concepts.

That said, even in the rare instances when things didn't end as I'd liked, the *Persuasion Sequence* demonstrated that everything possible was attempted to convince the subject to cooperate and that subsequent appropriate action was justified. Gary Klugiewicz, from Vistelar, often puts it this way: "The point is to at least look good, no matter how things end up."

A common example of the "looking good" benefit of the *Persuasion Sequence* might be when we are forced to *Take Appropriate Action* if patients or their family members are disruptive. In a few cases, physicians who were rightly advocating for their patients demanded answers for why their patients or their visitors were expelled. One conversation I once had with a provider went like this.

"You mean to tell me that you threw my patient's mother out of the hospital? Are you crazy?!" complained the doctor.

"Yes Ma'am, I did. I asked her to leave because she was disruptive and disturbing other patients on the unit."

"Well her kid just had surgery, for God's sake!" she said tersely.

"I understand that, doctor, but the kids on either side of her room also just had surgery." After using the *Redirections* tactic, I simply continued building context. "Their parents were complaining and one of the other kids was crying and upset because of that mother's behavior. Her actions were affecting not only her own child's recuperation, but that of other kids on the unit."

"Well couldn't you just have asked her to stop?"

"Oh I did just that, doctor. After I introduced myself, the next thing I did was ask her to stop yelling and cursing on the unit."

"What did she say?" she asked.

"She said 'F*** you!' loud enough for the whole hospital to hear," I replied.

"Okay, did you explain to her why she couldn't do that?" asked the doctor.

"Absolutely, I explained that she was frightening the other kids. I said I understood that she was angry and that I wanted to help her out."

"So....then what did she say?" asked the doctor, now in a much softer tone.

"Well, she said she didn't give a s**t about anyone else's kid and just kept threatening and cursing."

"Okay, so is that when you threw her out?" asked the doctor, sheepishly.

"No, not just yet. First I offered her a choice. I advised her that, if she stopped yelling, I would do whatever was in my power to help her out. I even offered to get a nursing supervisor and a quiet conference room we could use, so as not to disturb other patients."

"Really?" asked the doctor.

"Yep," I replied. "It's all in my report. But she just kept it up. She said she didn't want to discuss it and continued cursing and yelling at nurses and even at visitors as they walked on and off the unit."

At that, the doctor simply said, "Okay, okay I get it, you had no choice. That's when you threw her out."

"Nope," I said.

"Really? Why not?" she asked wearing a surprised expression.

"Because I wanted to give her an opportunity to reconsider. Like you say, her child just had surgery. So I asked if there was anything at all I could say to get her to stop causing a disturbance, and she yelled, "F*** you and this f***ing hospital!" at the top of her lungs. At that point I didn't have any choice but to escort her off the unit."

"Well, I guess you had no choice. So was my patient upset that his Mom was ejected from the hospital?" she asked.

"Well, he might have been and sometimes kids are upset when this happens. But in this case, I honestly think he was relieved."

So, as we've seen, the *Persuasion Sequence* not only makes us more effective communicators, but also effective behavior managers at the point of impact. We also are able to use it justify our actions.

Again, before using the *Persuasion Sequence* you must ask. Just as in the Big, Mean, Angry Biker story, we focus on behavior hoping to affect the attitude and generate voluntary cooperation. In the case of a gateway behavior like cursing in your facility, a *Persuasion Sequence* might need to be used after asking, "Sir, could I please ask you to stop cursing?" and not getting cooperation.

That is an example of an initial way you might approach things. Your expression should reflect concern and your tone of voice should be supportive and professional. In this way, you present your *on-stage face (Showtime Mindset)* to your patient. As Gary Klugiewicz often says, "the goal is to first create a reasonable doubt in their mind that you are not a jerk!" First impressions are everything. Once you've asked someone to do something, you should always offer the reason you're asking. Telling someone "it's the rules" or "because I asked you to" is a very natural response. But, as with most natural responses, they rarely work.

People want concrete reasons when you ask them to cooperate against their own judgment or when asking them to modify their behavior. "There are little kids around and they can hear you cursing" is a real-life explanation of why cursing, yelling, or threatening may be inappropriate. Also, trotting out your hospital's policies is rarely effective when not placed in proper sequence. Policies and laws can be effective in locking down context, however, after an explanation has first been offered. "Also, hospital policy does not allow cursing because this has to be a safe and appropriate environment for kids and families" is another way to set complete context for people who are resisting your attempts to address their behavior.

Once clear options are presented and people are given ample opportunity to cooperate, most will choose to go along with the program. For those who refuse, presenting them with their *Options*, or in other words *Choices*, is your next step. "Sir, we have a couple good options. You can stop cursing and I can try to help you out. I really want to help with whatever your situation is. But, if you insist on cursing in the hospital, I'll have to ask you to leave."

At this stage, it's very natural just to threaten, "If you don't stop, I'll call security." Threats never work. They are just challenges that beg to be taken up. If we were to start with the bad option first, the third step in the *Persuasion Sequence* always sounds like a threat. A bad example might be, "Sir, I can call security or you can just stop cursing and go about your day." Again, through training and practice, providers learn to offer the options in a professional and effective manner. By practicing saying prompters like, "We have some good choices," reminds us to start with the good options and avoid sounding threatening or authoritarian.

In the case below, a clinician sets limits while using a noticeably quiet volume and softer tone.

Clinician:	"Mr. Johnson, I know you're upset and I want to help. We have a couple good options. Just stop yelling and we can get to the bottom of what's bothering you, or let's step over to the conference room so we're not disturbing the other patients. But, if you insist on yelling and cursing in the clinic, I'll have to ask you to leave. Can you work with me?"
Mr. Johnson:	"You can't kick me out, I'm sick!," he replied urgently, but less loudly this time.
Clinician:	"I don't want you to leave. You need to be here with us. We want to get you well and start feeling better."
Mr. Johnson:	"Then help me." He asked now at a normal volume, following the clinicians' tone down to a safer place.
Clinician:	"We are helping you, Mr. Johnson. We checked your vitals and you're safe with us. Sit right here where we can keep an eye on you. The bathroom is right over there and you can't have any water right now, until we know exactly what is wrong with you or you could get sicker."
Mr. Johnson:	"Why can't you just see me now?" he pleaded.
Clinician:	"Because you are not the only sick person here.

Some of these people have been here longer and
a few of them are sicker than you are. Do you
want me to make them wait longer to see
you first?"

Mr. Johnson: "No."

Clinician: "Okay. I'm glad you understand. Honestly,
unless someone comes through that door with
a heart attack, we will see you within the hour.
Let's just keep our fingers crossed. Okay?"

Mr. Johnson: "Okay."

Non-verbal communication is just as important, if not more important, than what you say. Again, providers have the position of advantage in every situation where they are communicating with patients, families, or visitors, unless they choose by their actions to surrender it. In this case, the clinician gave clear options and empowered the patient to make the choice. She also locked down context by giving clear and concrete reasons why he couldn't be served immediately. Lastly, she modeled the behavior she wanted to see from her patient.

When we are challenged, our natural instincts are to match the tone and volume of the aggressor or clam up and shrink into a posture of submission. Neither approach is safe or productive. By "Reverse Yelling," we can reset the pace and volume of the conversation, causing the aggressor to follow us down to a quieter, calmer, safer level. *All behavior equalizes.* The person with the best communication skills sets the tone.

Reverse yelling is just another one of the psychomotor skills, like *Proxemics 10-5-2*, that practitioners of Vistelar's conflict management methodologies develop as they practice their skills in training. By sticking to the basics in scenario-based drills, they not only begin to master basic communications skills, they also build confidence that will guide them through conflict on the job, at home, and in their daily lives.

Chapter Seven
Is Everything Okay, Doctor?
When Word-Based Tactics Fail

"In any moment of decision, the best thing you can do is the right thing.
The worst thing you can do is nothing."

Teddy Roosevelt

The doctor arrived on the unit and suddenly found himself surrounded by angry nurses, demanding action. "You seriously need to talk to your patient's family!" the charge nurse said anxiously.

"Why, what's up?" said the surprised doctor. He was a good doctor and well liked by the nursing staff. He was used to nurses speaking their mind, as he was approachable, showed them respect, and genuinely valued their opinions.

"They've been arguing and fighting all day. Now they are refusing to leave and it's an hour after visiting hours! I was just about to call security!"

"No don't do that," pleaded the doctor. "If we call security, it might just make things worse. Let me see what I can do."

"Please, be my guest. They are sure not listening to us," complained the charge nurse, as the doctor headed towards his patient's room.

As he approached down the hallway, he could already hear several voices involved in a heated argument and the television turned up at a loud volume. While walking down the hall, he glanced into the other rooms with their doors open and saw other patients sleeping or quietly watching television. When he passed the patient room next door, he saw a woman standing in the doorway with an anxious expression on her face. Before he could say anything she asked, "Is everything okay, doctor?"

"I'm sure it is. I'm going to talk to them now," he answered in a reassuring tone.

The door to the problem patient's room was also open. He could see the patient lying in her bed, watching television and appearing undistracted by the chaos surrounding her. On either side of her bed were two men involved in a heated verbal exchange, while pointing and shaking their fists at each other. At their sides were two women, often chiming in by cursing and threatening the other in turn. Crowded together in a recliner were two little girls, who were also staring at the television intently, as if tuning out a familiar background noise. The doctor entered the room unnoticed. Without making a sound he quietly walked around to another chair in the opposite corner of the room and sat waiting for the family to settle down. The argument seemed to go on forever, but after a few minutes one of the men turned to leave and walked towards the door. He noticed the doctor sitting there. "Who the f*** are you, motherf*****?!" he demanded.

To that, the doctor stood up and said, "I'm this patient's physician and this has to stop!" Without answering, the man shoved the doctor back in his seat. When he attempted to stand again, the man's wife was on him immediately, slapping and scratching his face. When the other couple tried to intervene, an all out brawl was sparked. By the time security arrived, the doctor was already bruised, battered, and bleeding from his mouth. The patient and the two other little girls were crying and screaming in the back of the room.

Word-based tactics may fail, therefore effective conflict management demands that other viable options exist. Once you have exhausted all verbal options and reconciliation is no longer a feasible or safe option, *Taking Appropriate Action* is the next step in managing conflict. Every action you take is safety and circumstantially dependent. The need to take action may occur at any time during a conflict situation and not only after all possible verbal options have failed.

The need to *Take Appropriate Action*, including physical action when justified, can occur at any point during the *Persuasion Sequence* or at any other time, during contact with a challenging individual. The need for action occurs when the *Persuasion Sequence* is attempted but does not gain cooperation. If that happens, we can professionally and ethically invoke the right to take the appropriate action that fits the circumstances, such as expelling a visitor, calling the police, or discharging a patient.

The action you take should always depend on your personal safety and the safety of your patients, peers, staff, and visitors to your facility, in accord with the policies and procedures of your facility. Your particular institution may have regulations and policies that set your rules of engagement, which you should follow to the best of your ability. Those rules of engagement will always apply, as long as they don't conflict with your constitutional right of self-defense. Also, according to Joint Commission, Center for Medicare and Medicaid Services and OSHA standards, healthcare professionals have a responsibility to protect people under their care. In this day and age of rampant healthcare violence there are no more innocent bystanders!

Of course, the action you take must be reasonable in light of the circumstances and must be in line with your state's statutes concerning self-defense and the defense of others. When forced to defend others or ourselves, the force we use need not be a perfect selection, only a reasonable one. That is an important distinction, in that we are often forced to make a quick decision in uncertain and rapidly evolving circumstances. Although, ultimately, others will likely judge your use of force, the justification for its use is viewable only from *your* perspective, based on what you believed to be true at the time you act. Second-guessing and Monday morning quarterbacking are irrelevant except for the purposes of debriefing with an eye on improvement. Documenting, in writing, that you attempted the *Persuasion Sequence* will not only show that you performed to the best of your ability, it will protect you should legal and professional concerns arise.

That understood, you might not always have time to complete or even begin a *Universal Greeting* or *Persuasion Sequence*. Sudden assaults are rare, but do occur. The actions you take must be a trained technique that complies with your institutions rules of engagement or an untrained technique justifiable under the law according to the totality of the circumstances.

Healthcare professionals frequently deal with patients who suffer from trauma, brain injuries, psychiatric crises or who may be under the influence of drugs, alcohol, or general anesthesia. The failure to train healthcare staff in physical stabilization techniques is not only dangerous but also misguided. The option to never go "hands-on" does not exist in the real world, especially in the medical profession. Therefore, the responsibility for hospitals and clinics to train security and other hospital staff in physical stabilization techniques is a foregone conclusion. Through Vistelar's conflict management training program, clinicians, security, and support staff learn to forecast, non-escalate, disengage, de-escalate, and stabilize patients as necessary for the safety of both patients and providers.

An immediate safety concern is always a reason to *Take Appropriate Action* and a safety concern may develop at any time. You might be involved in a routine contact with a patient, employing the five approaches to showing respect, having a *Showtime Mindset,* going *Beyond Active Listening, Redirecting* verbal abuse and using the *Persuasion Sequence* but, despite your best efforts, safety concerns can arise.

Your ability to act depends on your understanding of tactical *Proxemics 10-5-2* techniques, i.e., proper distance, positioning and hand placement. It also depends on your ability to sense and recognize danger. The recognition of an immediate danger is based upon your ability to assess threat and the level of trust you place in your own instincts. Unfortunately, as we discussed, human beings are quick to dismiss their own instincts. Healthcare workers may be particularly impaired for two reasons: Violence Myth #7 ("Things aren't really that bad") and the false sense of security healthcare workers commonly develop. The following story is a good example.

A nurse had just finished her shift in the emergency room and decided to stop at an all night grocery on the way home. It was late and she didn't like to shop alone after dark but she didn't like waking up to an empty refrigerator either, so she dismissed her fears and stopped for some basic supplies.

She had a new car and didn't like to park it in crowded areas and risk door dings, so she parked it a little further away from the entrance. While walking across the parking lot she noticed someone driving slowly through the empty part of the large shopping center parking lot next door. She wondered to herself what they were looking for, as it seemed a little odd.

Once inside, she grabbed a cart and headed through the aisles. As always was the case, she started filling her cart with more than she'd originally intended to buy. While looking at some cosmetics, she noticed a man staring at her. As is true with most women, this wasn't a new experience for her. Many times in the past she had encountered the "creepy guy gaze." Being accustomed to being ogled on occasion, she just dismissed it and went on. But as the minutes passed, she noticed that the creepy guy kept turning up in every aisle she turned down. He would look her up and down, while obviously pretending to look at items on the shelves. He didn't have a cart and wasn't carrying anything either. He would just pick up an item or two, place them back on the shelves and nonchalantly follow her through the store at a distance.

Finally, when she turned down the next aisle he disappeared. Feeling somewhat relieved, she decided to forgo anymore shopping and head to the register. She looked around the store on her way up to the front, but couldn't catch sight of the creepy guy. Though she had been in that very same situation a few times before, she said it was my voice in her ear that gave her pause on that particular evening.

Two weeks prior to that evening, she attended one of my training sessions on the prevention and management of healthcare violence. In that training, I told the class to reclaim their natural sense of fear they had lost through their training and experience as providers. She said she particularly recalled my definition of a false sense of security, which comes from taking a risk several times and not getting hurt, then drawing a false conclusion that what you're doing is safe. It may not be the first ten times or even the first hundred times you do something dangerous that you get hurt or killed. It may happen on the one hundred and first time. Finally, she said she could hear me telling her to trust the little hairs on the back of her neck. On this night, the little hairs on the back of her neck were sticking straight up.

She said she knew what she had to do. That is, ask for help. Though she felt silly and embarrassed, she decided to tell the cashier about the creepy guy. In most cases we wouldn't judge someone else as being silly or weak for asking for help in these circumstances, but we still might judge ourselves harshly. In order to keep safe, sometimes we have to give ourselves a break for being cautious. If the worst did happen, both the victim and the Monday morning quarterback would be thinking that she *coulda, shoulda, woulda* asked for help.

"Excuse me," she said to the cashier. "I'm probably just being silly, but some creepy guy was staring at me in the store. Can someone walk me to my car or just watch to make sure I'm safe?"

"Oh dear!" said the cashier. "Don't feel silly, you were right to ask. Let me get the manager."

The assistant manager happened to be a man so they sent him. He was only too glad to walk the young nurse to her car, although it's not necessary for our support persons to always be men, because women can support us as well. As a matter of fact, I'll take a woman with some basic violence awareness and safety training over an untrained man any day. That said, he put on his jacket and valiantly escorted her out into the lot.

As they approached her car, she noticed that someone had parked next to her, all the way out there in the empty part of the lot. As the manager was kind of chatty, he didn't notice the look of fear on her face when she recognized it as the same suspicious looking car that was patrolling the lot when she first arrived at the store. While the manager kept talking about how he was only glad to escort her and wished more women would ask, curiosity overtook her judgment and she simply continued up to the parked cars.

When finally close enough, she looked though the windshield of the strange vehicle. Crouched down in the seat was the creepy guy, with his seat reclined far back enough to conceal his presence, but still give him a view of the lot. "That's him!" she shouted while pointing at the windshield. The startled manager started to approach the driver's side when creepy guy sat up, turned over the engine and sped away.

In the words of Bob Willis, "Threat assessment is the study of what human beings do before they assault you. In poker, experienced players can predict the future by noticing certain *"tells"* in the behavior or other players. Victims of assaults sometimes say that they knew they were about to be attacked but unfortunately chose not to act."

One of the things I've heard most often when debriefing victims of violent assaults is, "It came out of the blue!" Over my long career I've learned that's almost never the case. Usually, attackers tell their victims many times that an attack is coming, long before it actually happens. Sudden assaults are rare but do occur. That said, even in a sudden assault, the signs that violence is possible are usually present, in the form of pre-attack postures and other behavior patterns. Professionals, whether they are police officers or healthcare providers, need to always be on the job when in uniform. In the case of healthcare workers, they are on the job whenever they are wearing scrubs. It's not about being paranoid. It's about being relaxed but alert and then taking appropriate action when threats are identified, and when situations occur that require increased attention and caution.

STAMP and the *Gateway Behaviors of Violence* are two examples of behavior patterns that can reliably predict violent outcomes. Experienced professional fighters know what is about to happen, before it does. Another pattern of behavior that is related to *STAMP* is *pre-attack postures*.

Some pre-attack postures are dramatic, like the clenching of a fist. Others are subtle, like someone invading your personal space. There are early warning signs of rising emotion that can be heard, seen, or even felt. Increased tone and volume is easily recognized and should be respected, but murmuring under the breath or conspicuously ignoring attempts to communicate are also reliable signs of building tension. Angry expressions and threatening eye contact are also easily recognized. But the avoidance of eye contact or a blank expression, sometimes referred to as the thousand-yard stare, can be equally dangerous and too subtle to recognize by unaware providers who don't have their heads in the game. There are also body postures, such as shifting weight from one foot to another, shoulder shifting or "blading" the body at an angle. Increased tension can also be felt in the form of the *dead weight tactic*, when trying to lift or move a patient.

There is also your intuitive sense, built on your natural instincts and experience. If something seems out of the ordinary or threatening, it probably is. In those cases, take the most conservative approach, get help, and *Take Appropriate Action*. Don't wait for the attack to come. Instead, anticipate it and take measures to prevent it. Learning to disengage and using self-protection skills are essential for anyone working in healthcare.

The tipping point is often related to distance. As a preventive measure and assessment tool, we can employ the *Proxemics 10-5-2* tactic. Remember, if you are at ten feet, you can leave or not enter in the first place. Healthcare providers generally tend to go too fast, get too close, and say too much before they've made an *initial assessment of the scene*. Ironic, considering healthcare workers are constantly assessing patients.

In an environment crowded with people and crammed with equipment, such as many hospital settings, ten feet can seem like a huge distance. An ER exam room may be barely ten feet in depth! Still, our assessment often begins with the patient's chart and the circumstances of the patient's complaint. Armed with what we already know about a patient, we can continue our assessment by what we hear when approaching the room. So, that ten feet of evaluation space really begins in the hallway before we ever get to the room.

When we get to the door, we need to think of that space as the patient's current living space and not as an extension of our workspace. Whether the door is open or not, we need to knock on the door or doorframe, wait a few seconds, knock again, then open slowly if unanswered. Standing just outside the doorframe, we need to begin our evaluation. How many people are in the room? Is the patient present? How is everyone behaving? Are there any potential hidden danger areas, corners, curtains, and closed restroom doors?

In many hospital exam rooms, when we're standing in the doorway, we are already in the "five feet zone". That is the point at which we will need to *communicate or evade* if a threat is identified or an attack occurs. At five feet you could be fully involved in communicating with a patient or visitor, but ready to take necessary action to disengage from an attack. Through Vistelar's conflict management training program, providers learn effective stance and movement skills, such as sweep and escape, designed to maximize their ability to evade an attacker even when given one second or less to react. These skills are vital when you can't just turn your back and leave because of how vulnerable you've become and how quickly you can be assaulted at that range.

While communicating at five feet, providers can begin to form relationships that are incompatible with uncooperative and even violent behavior. Having a *Showtime Mindset* and using the *Universal Greeting* can set the tone for what happens next. It is also a point at which you can continue your threat assessment and determine if it's safe to approach your patient and operate. By operate, we mean examine and treat your patient. Once you've made the determination that the patient is ready to be approached and you've stated your intentions by use of the *Universal Greeting*, you can approach to within two feet. At that point, if we're threatened or attacked, we'll be required to defend ourselves and escape. But by assessing at ten feet and communicating at five feet, we've greatly reduced the possibility that an attack will occur. When we rush in too quickly, things are far more likely to go badly.

But what about those times when we're forced to *Take Appropriate Action* (*when word-based tactics fail*), either by calling the police, dismissing a patient, or even defending ourselves physically? Does taking action then constitute a failure on the part of providers?

On one occasion I was asked by a child protective service agency to assist with a family who was in foster care. The parents had court-ordered supervised visits with their biological children who were in the physical custody of a foster family. During the parent visits, the father would get confrontational with the foster parents and curse, yell, and otherwise behave inappropriately in front of the children. Even after repeated attempts to supervise visits by the foster parents and case managers, the father's behavior got progressively worse. Finally, he began to threaten the foster parents and caseworkers. Fearing for the safety of the children and agency staff members, the agency reached out for assistance.

I formulated a safety plan that first included a *risk assessment* that included a background check of the parents, a review of any records, a debriefing of the caseworkers, the orders from the court, and all the particulars of the case. A *risk assessment* is a gathering of information intended to predict possible threats from individuals or situations, based on what we know. Then I asked to meet with the parents prior to scheduling their next visit, in order to make a *threat assessment* by assessing their behavior. A *threat assessment* is an evaluation of behaviors and situations at the point of impact, based on what we can observe in the moment.

I scheduled the meeting in a secure setting at the agency, instead of the parents' home. When they arrived for our meeting, I greeted them with a *Universal Greeting*. "Good Afternoon, I'm Joel Lashley. I'm the security officer for the agency. It's a pleasure to meet you both. Can I ask your names?"

"Hello, we're Mr. and Mrs. Jackson," said the father. The mother didn't speak. In fact, she rarely spoke at all and only in response to questions.

"The reason we're here is so I could meet you both and discuss how I can assist you in having successful visits with your kids. May I see your paper work and identification?" They produced the items I requested and I escorted them to an office where we could talk privately.

As I expected, once we were alone the father became confrontational. He raised his voice and started cursing. He also denied threatening anyone or otherwise behaving badly during prior visits. He also demanded new caseworkers and that future visits be scheduled at his home. His wife kept her head down and seemed to just tune us both out. Using the *Persuasion Sequence*, I laid down some ground rules.

"Mr. Jackson, can I ask you to please lower your voice and stop cursing? We have to prepare for your visit with your children and this is the sort of behavior that we are concerned about."

"I can talk anyway I want! I'm a grown man!" he shouted.

"I'm not telling you how to speak anywhere else. But this is a place of business and it has to be an appropriate environment for children and families. So we don't allow any cursing, yelling, or threatening. The way you talk somewhere else is your own business, but not here. This is a private office," I explained in a concerned tone of voice and at a low volume.

"F*** that!" he replied while rolling his eyes, but also mimicking my calmer tone and volume, as he was already following me down to a calmer state of mind. But he was still cursing so I continued to set context.

"Mr. Jackson, I am here to make sure you can visit with your kids. I have determined that your behavior is threatening and uncooperative. If you refuse to cooperate with me, I'll have to cancel your visits until they can be re-evaluated by the court."

"You can't do that!" he said sternly, but still not yelling.

"We have two choices, Mr. Jackson, one good one and one bad one. The good one is, you can cooperate with me and agree to my terms. Then your visits with your kids will proceed on schedule. I will also write in my report for the court that you were cooperative. But if you refuse to hear me out and agree to my terms, I will report this conversation and recommend that future visits be terminated because you are too much of a risk to our staff and your children. Do you understand, Mr. Jackson?"

"Okay. I didn't curse or threaten anyone anyway," he replied.

"Well, that's good. Then you have nothing to worry about. I will be on hand for your next few meetings. If you're safe and cooperative with everything, I will testify to that on your behalf. I want to be on your side. Can you help with that? It's all up to you what happens next."

Mr. Jackson agreed to my terms, which were to meet with the caseworkers, immediately following our meeting. He also agreed to continue working with the assigned caseworkers. He also agreed not to yell, curse, or threaten during future visits and cooperate with staff direction and coaching.

The meeting with this family's caseworkers was scheduled immediately after my private meeting with the Jacksons. Much to my surprise, we would not be alone. When I led the Jacksons to the conference room for the next meeting, we found it to be crowded. Along with the caseworkers were their supervisor, the foster parents, the children's psychologist, the parents' attorney, and many other people I didn't recognize. With at least a dozen people crowded around the conference table, the meeting began.

Seated next to his attorney and seemingly emboldened by his presence, Mr. Jackson looked poised for a fight. As soon as one of the caseworkers attempted to open the meeting, he interrupted her, saying, "I don't want to hear anything out of you! I don't want you on my case anymore!"

"Mr. Jackson," I interjected. "We just talked about this. Do you want to proceed or should I just cancel this meeting now?"

"I'm sorry." He replied and sat quietly. The look on everyone's face was priceless as his immediate cooperation was totally unexpected.

At times during the meeting, Mr. Jackson would raise his voice or drop an f-bomb. At those junctures I would just say, "Mr. Jackson", and he would apologize and settle down. On another occasion, he caught himself, apologized, and stopped before I could say anything.

After a few curious looks from his attorney, the meeting continued swimmingly. Then after two hours of hard negotiation and discussion, Mr. Jackson received news he wasn't prepared for. The visits would continue at the agency until further notice and the children would remain in foster care. After hearing that, he blew up. "You f***ing b***h!" he shouted while lunging across the table at the caseworker. Before he could reach her I was on him. The security officer and I took him out into the common area where he continued to fight. Ultimately we handcuffed him and called the police to take custody.

While we waited for the police to arrive, Mr. and Mrs. Jackson wept softly. Finally, I addressed the father while we waited. "Mr. Jackson, it's really none of my business now. I know this must be hard. But you have to understand. If you keep behaving like this, they will never give you your kids back."

To that, he looked me in the eye and asked, "Really?"

For the first time, the mother looked up and spoke without being spoken to. She looked directly at her husband and said, "Do you get it now?"

After the police came and took Mr. Jackson away, I directed Mrs. Jackson to the bus stop and went home. All of the other people from our meeting had already left. I was certain that complaints would soon pile in from the agency and the parent's attorney about what a disaster the meeting had been. Sure enough, by the next morning my voicemail and email were both flooded with messages. However, these responses weren't at all what I expected. They were filled with praise about the meeting and requests to continue having me supervise future meetings. The caseworkers in particular, said they had never accomplished as much with this client at a single meeting, as they always had to be cancelled within a few minutes. The agency also wanted my help with other difficult cases.

In every encounter, things may not go as expected. Outcomes can even appear different to different people. But as Mr. Klugiewicz often says, "We must have a pre-planned, practiced response so that no matter where things end up, we always look good."

Joel Lashley

Chapter Eight
Shouldn't Somebody Say Something?
Bystander Mobilization

"When bad men combine, the good must associate; else they will fall one by one, an unpitied sacrifice in a contemptible struggle."
Edmund Burke

The man had arrived at the walk-in clinic three hours ago and had already asked twice how much longer he was going to have to wait to see a doctor. He left work at lunchtime to finally seek medical care, because nothing he had tried over the past three days seemed to be helping his abdominal distress. He tried to get in to see his family doctor, but no appointments were available that day, only adding to his anxiety. His wife kept calling his cell every 30 minutes or so, to check on him and remind him that their daughter had a soccer game that afternoon. Finally, he was beginning to boil over.

"So what's taking so long? Aren't you at a *walk-in* clinic?" she said sarcastically. "I thought you were supposed to just walk-in and get treated right away. Isn't that the point?"

"How should I know? They're busy, I guess," he replied.

117

"What about Ashley's game?" she asked.

"I'm sick! Do you really think I can go to that game tonight!" he shot off angrily, feeling hurt by her indifference to his ailment.

"Well, I at least need you home to watch the other kids, so I can take her. It's an important game!" she shouted back.

"I just told you I'm sick!" he shouted into the phone. "All of her g*****n games are important! Why don't you just take the other kids with you?"

"I'm the assistant coach! How the hell am I supposed to watch them and coach at the same time?" she fired back.

"Oh, okay then. I'll just leave and be right home!" he replied. "And thanks for the concern! I could have f***ing stomach cancer for all you know!"

The receptionist made every effort not to make eye contact, with the angry man on the phone and just went busily about her job. Then a nurse stepped out from the back and handed her some forms to process, paying no more attention to all the shouting and cursing then if it had been the hum of an air conditioner. To her, it was just another familiar background noise of the workplace, like the beeping of an I.V. pump. Finally, a lab tech stuck her head into the reception area and asked, "What's going on?"

"He's fighting with his wife," whispered the receptionist. The lab tech scanned the room and saw an elderly couple stand up. With his wife close on his heels, the elderly man scooted quickly behind his walker, intent on creating as much space as possible between themselves and the angry man. Some patients crawled deeper into their well-worn magazines, while others looked on disapprovingly. Others struggled to distract their children's attention from the angry man's shouting and profane language.

"Shouldn't somebody say something?" asked the lab tech.

"Tell his nurse," replied the receptionist. The lab tech went back to the treatment area and quickly spotted the physician's assistant and one of the nurses huddling together over a medical record. "Do you hear that guy yelling out there?" she asked with a puzzled expression.

"I hear him," said the physician's assistant. "Did the receptionist say anything to him?"

"Doctor Jenkins should probably say something to him," chimed in the nurse.

"He's kind of busy right now for that," replied the PA.

"In that case," replied the nurse, "I'll try and get one of these rooms cleared out as soon as possible so we can get that guy back here. He sounds like he's just angry about the wait."

"Good idea," said the PA. "Hopefully that will shut him up."

Hurt and angry, due to his wife's badgering and uncaring attitude, the angry man hung up on her mid-sentence. Then he stood and walked urgently up to the receptionist, yelling, "What the hell is taking so f***ing long!"

For the first time she looked up and made eye contact with the angry man, simply saying, "I'll tell your nurse that you're waiting."

Scenarios like the above are played out in waiting rooms, treatment areas, and patient rooms all day long, in hospitals and clinics all around the world. The United States isn't the only place where people fight in hospitals. China, India, Australia, France, England, Germany, Mexico, Sudan, on every continent, in every country, in every city, it seems like clinical violence is on the rise. Why?

Like I said before, when most people go to a hospital they arrive with several problems. Health problems, family problems, professional problems, substance abuse problems, and financial problems that are all directly or indirectly connected to their medical issue. That understood there are definitely other issues that generate violence in the hospital setting.

The most obvious issue is that stress is a factor in treatment. Fear, pain, and disruption of daily routine all conspire to push patients from stress into crisis. When healthcare workers fail to train and apply the principles of non-escalation, they often end up ensuring that violent incidents occur. Violent incidents that could have been avoided, with the right training and direction.

Secondly, domestic violence is more prevalent in hospitals than in other workplaces for both patients and staff. Primarily because families interact closely in hospitals for long periods, while under stress. As a result, arguments between family members are a common security issue in hospitals. When healthcare professionals fail to manage the early stages of conflict, i.e., gateway behaviors, violence often results. Again, violence that is both predictable and avoidable!

Also, more than three out of four providers in hospitals, clinics, and sub-acute facilities are women and almost nine in ten home healthcare workers are women. Women are more likely than men to be the victims of sexual assault, sexual harassment, and intimate partner violence. Often, issues connected with stalking and intimate partner violence spill over into the workplace, because the workplace is the one place in most people's lives where they can reliably be intercepted. You can change your shopping habits, social habits, and even meet friends and family in neutral places when trying to avoid stalkers and ex-domestic partners. You can even change your church, your friends and where you live. But the one geographical constant in most people's lives is where they work.

Hospitals and clinics must prepare for this reality, by enacting vigorous domestic violence prevention programs not just for patients but also for staff. These programs should include: training staff to recognize potential threats and assess risk; creating a supportive and respectful atmosphere where potential victims feel safe to report threats to their personal safety; training security to conduct threat assessments on reported issues (in the absence of a professional security department, local police departments can be contacted directly to assess risk); finally, training to formulate safety plans in order to keep the potential victim and other staff members safe.

Anyone can be a victim of stalking and sexual assault, including men. Anyone can also end up a victim of intimate partner violence. When these issues are drawn into the workplace, as they often are, we must prepare to recognize and avoid them.

The presence of narcotics is another issue that increases violent incidents in hospitals. Emergency rooms sometimes attract drug-seekers attempting to feign illnesses in order to acquire prescription narcotics. People under the influence of narcotics seek treatment in emergency rooms in large numbers as well. Rarely, robberies and thefts of narcotics occur in hospitals, as do drug diversion attempts by staff addicted to narcotics. Confrontations resulting from drug diversions cannot only harm a patient's well being but create conflict between staff members.

Insufficient resources of psychiatric care in society are also a big contributor to the level of violence in healthcare. As previously discussed, people with drug and alcohol problems wind up frequently in our emergency rooms. Also, people with all sorts of psychiatric disorders are funneled to emergency rooms as their only resource for care and critical intervention. Levels of brain-based disorders such as Alzheimer's, dementia, and autism are at record levels and increasing, all at a time when hospitals have all but closed down their in-patient psychiatric units and community crisis centers are in short supply.

As a society, we made the grand decision to close all of the sweeping institutions and psychiatric facilities that once housed hundreds of thousands of psychiatric patients and, for many reasons, that was a good thing. The problem is we didn't have a plan B! For far too many people with psychiatric and brain-based disorders the last stop is a prison or jail. And far too many of those are routed directly from the emergency department of a hospital.

Forensic patients are another issue that is largely ignored in hospitals, by both hospital administrators, police, and corrections professionals. A hospital is the only place—other than a courtroom—where society's prisoners interact directly with the public. If a prisoner needs a haircut, he goes to the prison barber. But if he needs emergency care, surgery, dialysis, or some other medical intervention, he may likely be sitting right next to you in a public waiting room. Not surprisingly a hospital is one of the more common places where prisoner escapes occur, yet most police departments and corrections facilities do little if any training in how to manage prisoners in hospitals.

In the wake of all the incidents involving prisoners in public hospitals and clinics, the medical profession must finally partner with the law enforcement profession to properly manage forensic patients because, whether we like it or not, public medical facilities are often an extension of their local jail or prison. Police and corrections officers must train to properly manage prisoners in the healthcare setting. Policies and procedures must be developed by medical facilities and providers trained for the proper management and security of forensic patients as well. This is a very real problem that results in injuries, escapes, and deaths each year. They are injuries, escapes, and deaths that could be avoided with proper training and direction.

The last reason on this list is violence attracts violence. People injured by violence require treatment at hospitals. Seems like an obvious statement, but it's a reality that is largely ignored. America is arguably the most violent developed nation on earth. Among the nations of Europe and next to our neighbor Canada, we have no peer in our predilection to violence. In fact, you have to go to a third world country to surpass our levels of violence. All the gun and gang violence sends both children and adults to emergency rooms in big cities every day. Most everyone who has worked for long in an urban emergency room has seen multiple gunshot victims in a single day. And all that violence has baggage.

Whenever a gunshot victim is admitted to a hospital, police and family members fill waiting rooms and even treatment areas. Almost always bring in family members struggling with grief and crisis. Sometimes, those family members are bent on revenge. It also can bring gang members attempting to support victims and who may also be seeking revenge. When victims of gang related violence survive and are being treated in hospitals, the potential exists for bringing members of an opposing gang who are seeking to finish the job.

So what is there to do? Just as in the example at the beginning of this chapter, no one can decide who is responsible to act. The bystander effect is a well established phenomenon demonstrating that the more people that are present in an emergency, the less likely an individual will take action. Therefore, we must begin by making it clear that it is everyone's responsibly to do something when a dangerous condition occurs. Then we have to give them the authority to act. In hospitals, when people act out, staff may feel even less able to intervene because of the mythology of healthcare violence discussed in chapter two. In training, we need to demonstrate how violence occurs and train staff to intervene as a team.

Step one in bystander mobilization training is to notice that a dangerous or potentially violent condition exists. By understanding the *Gateway Behaviors of Violence*, *STAMP* behavior, and other indicators, providers can begin to recognize the signs of violence. Secondly, we need to assume responsibility. Again, this is supported by policies, procedures and training that remove barriers to proper action by all staff members. This is the primary responsibility of leadership, meaning physicians and administrators, because staff needs permission and authority to act. Then providers need training to make safe assessments, in order to choose the proper type and level of intervention. Should they step in themselves or get help first? Or should they just step back and call security or police? Once the type and level of intervention is chosen, they need communications training in order to make an effective and safe intervention.

Vistelar consultant and bystander mobilization expert, Jill Weisensel, puts it this way, "Bystanders generally know right from wrong, but are unsure of how or when to take action to prevent a situation from getting worse. Most people think that intervention strategies require some drastic form of physical intervention; however, many appropriate strategies have very little to do with physical defense, and have everything to do with communication skills."

All that aside, providers must understand when personal intervention isn't the safest or best options and when to seek help. In the event of physical contact, personal defense options will be required. These skills can only be developed through dedicated instructor led training.

Nothing can replace well-trained providers and security personnel when one is seeking to prevent and mitigate violence in hospitals and clinics. But even a well-trained staff needs policies and procedures that are designed to prevent violence. Policies regarding the securing of narcotics, victim support, visitation procedures, the management of forensic prisoners and physical security procedures all work together to reduce the levels of violence in a hospital. But if we're not all on the same page, we're going to continue to struggle with all this violence. The importance of communications skills and non-escalation/violence prevention skills, that includes bystander mobilization training, cannot be overestimated.

Chapter Nine
If You Didn't Write It Down, It Never Happened
Review and Report

"Trust is a beautiful thing, but it has no place in police work."
Gary T. Klugiewicz

After any incident, no matter how large or small, it is important to review and report so mistakes aren't repeated and good practices are identified. Reviewing an incident will improve future performance and build consistency. Report writing protects you and your employer from speculation and documents your professionalism. Whenever we're looking back to a past incident in an effort to justify our performance, if we failed to file a report in the first place, as far as everyone else is concerned, it never happened that way. Report writing is a chore and it may also be human nature to try to forget about unpleasant experiences, but it is an essential task that enables us to advance and learn. A serious incident requires that a reconstructive effort is made and an analysis performed.

There will never be two incidents or two perspectives that are exactly the same. Even if you aren't the only person there, you are still the only one who has the information required to relate the incident as you saw it and experienced it. Others may critique your work, second-guess you and maybe even blame you, so it is important to articulate your perspective skillfully and detail exactly what you knew at the moment you took action.

Articulation is a skill that, ironically, many human service professionals lack. Complicating the situation, eyewitness testimony, video evidence and pictures are very likely tainted, because they were generated from a "passive" location, resulting in different perspectives and points-of-view than yours. In some cases, the very video recordings you thought would save you turn out to be worthless. Or worse yet, end up representing you in an ambiguous or even negative light. Any evidence that is subject to interpretation—such as video evidence—is viewed through the lens of a subjective observer. Photographic images and video evidence are also questionable for technical reasons, as these media are subject to distortion and confined to two dimensions.

Eyewitness testimony is often unreliable, because human memory can be affected by stress, emotion, and the passage of time. Many recent high profile incidents have demonstrated that lots of people can witness an incident and all report different versions of the event. Despite any evidence and others testimony, you will generally have only one chance to tell your story. Therefore, it must be truthful according to your best recollection and it must be well done.

Children's Hospital of Wisconsin has recently renewed focus on that very important aspect. Developing a culture incompatible with violence requires that intelligence information is generated and that providers are held accountable to take action. Once a violent incident or a condition that can result in violence is identified, whatever is learned enhances the ability to prevent future violence. Accountability will demand that we learn from the past and implement policies and procedures that have proven themselves in the field. Providers will ultimately learn awareness regarding the patterns leading to violence and utilize avoidance strategies and intervention tactics that they can apply early in the cycle of violence often preventing even the possibility of conflict.

The first question that may be asked is, "Whose responsibility is it to document a risk or violent incident?" Is it the provider, their supervisor, an administrator, the security department, risk management, or a law enforcement agency? The fact is that many of those people may be involved, but it is first and foremost your responsibility. You may be required to generate a written report, respond to a supervisor's questions, submit to an interview or even testify at a hearing.

The idea of writing a report or testifying in court terrifies many people, especially ones who are not called upon frequently to do so. Some may even fear that they are being accused of being involved in some way or otherwise suspect. Employers in the healthcare profession must first make it clear to providers and support staff that they have permission to report and take proper action when violent conditions occur. Then, and only then, can they make clear the expectation that everyone take action, no matter what their role is in the organization. Then healthcare facilities need to train providers how to identify unsafe conditions. Finally, they need to train staff how to take proper action, up to and including report writing. Only then can they truly begin to hold people accountable for their actions or inactions.

There are many levels of conflict in any incident. The first conflict might be either a violent incident that you just experienced or a condition of risk that you just identified, but it doesn't necessarily end there. A second conflict may involve justifying your actions to your peers, your employer, and in rare cases the police or in court.

Finally, we are often conflicted ourselves about whether we did the right thing. All these conflicts are related but require different abilities on your part. Having your "ducks in a row" is critical and fortunately well within your ability, especially because you have hopefully embraced the contents of this book. Vistelar's conflict management methodologies are a "system" that gets us through the incident and all the subsequent related conflicts.

Now that we have established that it is everybody's responsibility to review and report violent incidents and unsafe conditions, there are some ground rules. The first one of these rules is the "is everybody ok?" rule. Debriefing an incident is important but the welfare of those involved is the first priority. Forcing articulation or conducting an interview prematurely will not only harvest poor information, it will alienate everyone to the system and reduce future performance. Before debriefing can begin, the incident has to be stabilized and everyone involved must be both physically and emotionally safe.

The United States is currently dealing with renewed fallout of individuals struggling with Post Traumatic Stress Disorder, from the ranks of military and law enforcement personnel who have not been effectively reintroduced back into a "normal" social environment. Suicides are endemic in both the military and law enforcement communities because the physical and psychological welfare and normalization of these heroic people was too long an afterthought. A whole generation of Vietnam veterans returned to the demands of re-socialization without a general concern for their individual welfare; resulting in more of them dying by suicide, and drug and alcohol abuse, than by enemy fire. No matter the level and type of conflict, the initial step of the debriefing process must be to ask the question, "Is everyone okay?"

The next stage is to develop an emotionally safe environment. Debriefing is not intended to be an interrogation or fault finding mission, but a fact finding mission intended to report the truth to the best of our ability and to improve future performance. The purpose is to make us better the next time. Subsequent remedial measures are a legally recognized concept. If something could have been done better, it's important for everyone involved to take note and improve. Admitting our mistakes, while looking towards improvement, does not constitute an admission of liability. It's the way we learn as an institution and demonstrate our commitment to safety.

Debriefing also isolates what we did well and causes us to repeat good tactics and techniques. It is not about where we failed, because previously our experience was lacking, but where we can now, based on this incident, improve our performance. It is about what we have learned. The fact is that no one starts their day trying to figure out where they can screw up! The difference between a mistake and liability is reputation. The first time our performance is lacking, is usually because of our lack of experience; but the second and subsequent time our performance is lacking, is likely because we didn't debrief and bother to learn and seek improvement.

After the initial debrief, which is usually a discussion, the next stage may be an actual re-creation or walk through. After a traumatic event we may not remember things well. Human memory is complex and consists of recall and recollection. Recall is what we initially remember. Recollection, or associative memory, sometimes requires sensory stimuli to prompt memory. Going back to the scene, seeing objects or the environment, smelling the smells and touching or feeling things may fill gaps in memory. The walk-through is an attempt to identify the totality of the circumstances and the truth. Sometimes, during and after a traumatic event, focus becomes limited. By expanding our focus the totality of the circumstance becomes clearer.

Recognition memory completes the mosaic of an event by adding the feeling and emotion to your experience and training. It reflects not only on the objective but the subjective aspect—not just the cognitive but the emotional and psychological aspects as well.

Emotional intelligence is a known and recognized entity. It is an important part of our decision making process and must be a part of recounting an event. How were you feeling at the time you took action? How may your state of mind have affected your actions? Were you in fear for your safety or the safety of others when you took action? Did you perceive that there was no other recourse? Did you attempt other means to stabilize the situation? These aren't questions that seek blame. Instead, they are questions that clarify our intentions and often justify our course of action.

When necessary a debriefing can be accomplished by interviewing the individual players in an incident. In the busy task-driven environment of healthcare, group debriefings can be very difficult to pull off. Still, when individual players can share their perspectives together, better recall and safety planning becomes possible. That said, some people might be inappropriate to include in-group debriefings. This might include, of course, suspects, victims, patients, and visitors who may have been witnesses.

It is important to understand what you perceived but also what others perceived. These individual and collective parts help assemble a clearer picture of an incident. None of us are looming above an incident and watching it in its totality; we all observe varying parts of the entire event. The truth can only be assembled though a collaboration between the different observers, because no one person saw the whole thing. It may also be helpful to have trainers, risk managers, corporation attorneys, supervisors and other experts present. Not with the intention of spinning the story, but to make sure all bases are covered and that no element is overlooked.

Total recall and a search for the truth is an evolving process. Even if some people are less than truthful, the members of a debriefing group will ferret out and identify discrepancies. When preparing to debrief an incident, get yourself ready by going through the strategies, tactics and techniques taught in this book. An incident is less like a photograph and more like a movie. When filing your report, your articulation must describe how this event evolved and all the influences that exerted pressure upon it. Ultimately you are the one who makes the reader walk in your shoes.

When necessary, creating some emotional distance from an incident can allow you to achieve some professional detachment. Harry Dolan, retired Chief of Police of Raleigh, North Carolina, uses what he calls the 24-hour rule. Overnight, anger or fear may subside. After a short time to decompress, improved recall and collaboration may result.

Although it's often important to capture information from witnesses and victims while it's fresh and people are available, when debriefing other responders you can take a brief pause, step back, and cool off, so better information can rise to the surface. Questions like, Why were you there? What did you see? What threat assessment did you do? Did you use a *Universal Greeting*? Did you use the *Persuasion Sequence*? Did you use *Redirections*? What dangers were present? Did you employ a pre-planned and practiced response? Did you follow through properly after the event? Did you learn anything from this incident? Perhaps three of the most important questions you will be asked are: Is everybody okay? Did you respond as trained? If not, did you respond in a manner that was justified under the circumstances? All these questions become clearer when we have cool heads.

When analyzing an incident with an eye on improving future performance, we should always consider the closure principle: Did we leave the people we were dealing with in better condition than when we found them at their worst? How were they ultimately safer because of your presence and your actions? Look at the "big picture" and consider how others were affected by your intervention. Did they benefit from your intervention? Were they negatively impacted in anyway? Is there anything left to do post-incident? Although the incident itself may have been negative, opportunities for positive outcomes should never be squandered because we failed to review and report.

Chapter 10
Good Doc, Bad Doc
Point Of Impact Crisis Intervention

"A gentle answer turns away wrath, but a harsh word stirs up anger."
Proverbs 15:1

The dispatch center advised all units that a combative patient had just arrived at the emergency department via ambulance. I was the security supervisor on duty and responded from another building across campus. The rest of the security team was closer, all were experienced and well trained so I wasn't overly concerned, during the drive over. By the time I arrived, I could already hear a commotion coming from the exam room where the patient had been wheeled in. When I poked my head in I saw a tall, young, athletic man spitting, cursing, and struggling against the EMTs' tie-on cloth restraints.

The patient had taken an overdose of prescription medications and alcohol. He was also very strong and obviously feeling no pain. The EMTs had "packaged" him on their gurney in the *swimmer's position*, with one hand tied above his head in an effort to restrict his mobility. The swimmer's position isn't the safest position for

133

a patients' body or psychiatric well being, making it inappropriate for hospital use. Although medical-surgical cloth restraints are commonly used in hospitals for combative patients, we needed to get them off of him.

Medical-surgical type cloth restraints are fine for temporality immobilizing the arm of a confused patient, who is unconsciously pulling at an I.V. line or scratching a wound site; but they are unpadded, rough in texture, and ill-fitting, making them hard on a combative patients' circulation and skin integrity. We also needed to get both of his arms down at his side, as it makes a patient feel less vulnerable, especially if they have a history of violent or sexual trauma. It also places the patient in the optimal position to provide care and reduces strain on their muscles and joints. Therefore, the security team was preparing to transfer him to a hospital gurney and apply a five-point restraint kit specifically designed for combative hospital patients.

They were doing a nice job and had enough help, so I simply stood by, ready if needed.

Suddenly, a young resident physician walked in, while the nurses quietly prepared their I.V. lines and the security officers deftly continued stabilizing the combative patient. "Now you knock that off right now!" she shouted. "We're trying to help you, so just lay there and be quiet!"

The patient took a few seconds to process what the young physician had just said. Then suddenly, he exploded. "F*** you, you f***ing stupid b****!" he shouted. Since the security team was in the middle of a transfer to the restraint kit, he managed to free one leg and kick over an I.V. pump. He thrashed and kicked wildly and the security team had to manually stabilize the patient, while the nurses froze or backed away. Just as I stepped forward to help, the curtains to the exam room flung open.

An older surgeon passing by overheard the commotion and decided to see if he could help. He asked at the nurses' station for the patient's chief complaint and his name. What he did next was truly remarkable. As soon as he entered the room, he asked, "Who doesn't need to be in here right now?" He didn't have to ask twice, because every nurse and the young resident stepped out of the room immediately. Then he switched off the overhead examination lights and swung them out of the way. Then he said to all of us on the security team, "Okay guys, just stay quiet and I'll do all the talking." While we continued to apply the restraint kit, the doctor began to speak directly to the patient.

"Hello John," he said. "I'm Dr. Washington." The doctor spoke in a normal volume. He also spoke slowly and clearly, using a calm and reassuring tone. As he spoke, I think everyone on the security team started to feel their own tension diminish. After a brief pause, he continued talking to the patient who was still struggling and cursing. "John, you are in the hospital. You took too many pills." The doctor paused again, giving time for the patient to cognitively process this new information—information that was obvious to everyone, except perhaps the patient himself. "John, we have to help you or you will get very sick," he continued. "Please stop fighting and let us help you. You are safe with me here. I promise."

At that point, you could hear the patient *out-gas* with a large exhale, as the tension fell away from his body. At each step, the doctor coached the patient into submission. "John, we are going to put these around your wrists to keep you still. We have to work fast, so please don't struggle." At that, he nodded to signal us to continue applying the restrain kit.

Dr. Washington and the patient started to have a conversation, while the nurses were slowly reintroduced into the scene. "This nurse is going to poke your arm because we need to get some medicine in you fast. Please hold still." If the nurses and security officers were too loud or talking unnecessarily, he would "shush" us, reminding us to keep down the chatter. Soon, the patient was stable, being lavaged, and supported by his family.

When Dr. Washington turned to leave, I followed him. "Doc, you have a second?" I asked.

"Sure," he replied.

"That was nice work in there. Thanks for your help."

"No problem, glad I could help," he replied.

"You should teach that technique to the doctors in training. Where did you learn it?" I asked.

"It comes with experience. I'm not sure you can teach it," he replied.

"That's too bad," I said, "because if you could teach it, these other doctors wouldn't have to wait twenty years to learn it." With that he nodded, smiled, and left.

Over the years I've seen scores of *Crisis Interventions*. Sadly, most of them ended badly. One thing I've learned is that natural language is disastrous. None of us really know what to do in a crisis, unless we're trained or smart enough to learn from experience. That is, if we are lucky enough to learn from experience before getting hurt. Good training takes others' experience and transfers it to someone else. We can only accomplish that through instructor led, experiential, scenario-based training.

I've been trained in several different types of *Crisis Intervention* techniques and "service recovery" models that either fell flat on their face when I needed them most or even made things worse! It's true that human behavior is too unpredictable for all communications techniques to work in every case and on every person. That said, perhaps a method could be devised that is reliable enough and *flexible* enough to work on most people under most circumstances.

When customers, clients, and patients are wronged, we need to quickly repair that professional relationship. Sometimes we make mistakes and if we want to keep our customers, we better get good at making amends. One of the more common models of service recovery is the LEAD model. LEAD stands for Listen, Empathize, Apologize, and Do something. The first three words in the acronym are the same, no matter where you find them. In some places, the D might stand for "Deliver" or "Do the right thing". In service recovery situations, it really works! LEAD is used everywhere from hospitals to airlines and it gets results. Fewer complaints and fewer lost clients. But if LEAD is the only trick in your bag, what are the possible consequences? Imagine the following situation.

A patient is yelling and cursing in his room, about his television going out and throws a bedpan out into the hallway. His nurse runs to the room to see what's wrong. Armed with her LEAD training, she's confident she can handle the situation.

LISTEN: "Mr. Gordon, what's the matter?"

                       "My TV went out, g******it!" says the patient.

EMPATHIZE: "That's awful. You must be bored to death."

                       "If I don't get a TV in here right now I'm going to sue!"

APOLOGIZE: "I'm sorry Mr. Gordon. I'll call right away."

                       "You better. I've had it with this f***ing hospital."

DELIVER: "Can I get you a snack or some more coffee while you wait?"

                       "Just tell them a**holes to hurry the f*** up with my TV!"

In this scenario, all of the elements of LEAD were applied, but what did it accomplish? On the surface it appears that it only accomplished one thing. It trained the patient to curse and yell at his nurse whenever he wants something, because in this hospital yelling and cursing gets results.

Again, LEAD is a good service recovery model. People have the right to complain and get angry when things go badly. But they don't have the right to engage in the gateway behaviors that lead to violence. By training providers to use *Beyond Active Listening*, we have much more flexibility, including the ability to set limits on gateway behavior.

LISTEN:	"Mr. Gordon, what's the matter?"
	"My TV went out, g******it!" says the patient.
EMPATHIZE:	"I heard you all the way down the hallway. I can hear you are upset. I know it's been a rough day for you," replied the nurse.
	"Listen, b***h, this is bulls***. If I don't get a TV in here right now, I'm going to sue this f***ing place!"
PARAPHRASE:	"So you're saying you are this angry and threw a bed pan out in the hall because your TV isn't working?" asked the nurse.
	"No, d***it. Not just that. My leg hurts like hell and you won't give me any more meds!" replied the patient.
SUMMARIZE:	"Okay, Mr. Gordon. I'm glad you said some thing. Your doctor said you are maxed out on your usual pain meds for today. But there are other things we might be able to try. I'll call her and see what she says, but please stop yelling, cursing and throwing things.

I want to help you and I will. But you are frightening the other patients. There are kids and elderly people around. Can you work with me?"

"Yeah, I'm sorry," replied the patient.

It's okay, Mr. Gordon. I know you're hurting. Let me go try and do something to help. I'll be back as soon as I can. In the meantime, I'll have someone bring you an icepack and we can also try to reposition you a little."

Communication models will often fail if they are inflexible. Inflexible in the sense that they fail to mine for important information, set limits on unwanted behaviors, and formulate care plans and safety plans for moving forward. Also, communication skills aren't just a series of steps; they are psychomotor skills that must be developed through training.

In healthcare, law enforcement, and any human service work, we don't just deal with dissatisfied customers. We deal with people in genuine crisis and those suffering from mental illness. There are times when people will exhibit gateway behaviors when in psychiatric crisis. On these occasions, we need to focus on the crisis and the behavior. Just as in the example at the beginning of this chapter. So what exactly did the surgeon do in the former example? The first thing he did was, reduce stimulation.

People in crisis act-out for a reason—not because of a diagnosis. This is also true of the patient with the broken television. Though his broken television may have been the last straw, the real reason he acted-out was because of his pain. This is a very common scenario in medicine. But the man in restraints acted-out because of the ingestion of narcotics and alcohol, so how did the surgeon get to the root of his problem? First we have to manage the sources of stimulation and frustration that all people in crisis have in common. The first of these commonalities is *external stimulation*.

The primary sources of external stimulation are light, sound, and the human presence. The first thing the surgeon did was to remove all unnecessary people from the room. He allowed the security team to stay because they were essential for the safety of the patient and himself. That said, he managed their presence by instructing them not to talk. This is the *one voice* concept.

Healthcare is a labor-intensive profession. Anyone who has been to a cardiac code call, or "code blue" as it's commonly referred to, understands that. I've seen as many as twenty or more people crammed into a small patient room during a medical emergency with doctors, nurses, respiratory techs, and others all talking at once. I've also heard doctors struggling sometimes to get things under control by yelling something like, "Everyone just shut up!" Though that usually works, hearing doctors struggle to maintain order during a medical emergency is not very reassuring to the patient, the staff, and especially any family members within earshot. By training everyone to use the *one voice command*, we can restore voice discipline at the scene quickly, effectively, and professionally.

The human voice is one of the strongest forms of *external stimulation*. One voice equals communication. Two voices is just noise. Three voices equal chaos that is just another source of adrenaline to a subject in crisis. People in crisis abhor strange voices and sound. Unfortunately, healthcare providers and first responders hate silence. We all want to talk because we all want to help. The *one voice* command is a tool we can use at the scene to restore voice discipline in these situations as well. If everyone was trained in the one voice concept, it's possible that the surgeon in the example may not have even needed to restore voice discipline, because everyone would have already understood that dynamic. But at very least, by stating loudly and clearly "One voice!" he could have accomplished the same goal.

He also removed unnecessary harsh lighting, by moving the examination lights out of the way and turning down the remaining lights — another way to *reduce stimulation*. We don't need to have things dark, but lowering lights to a safe level is an effective tactic.

What he also did was *separate and support* the patient. Too many people at the scene, unnecessarily providing stimulation to a patient, is a common problem. By removing non-essential personnel, he managed that problem. Often, when people are in crisis, we need support for our own safety, but having support staff out of sight can go a long way to calming subjects down. With that in mind, he kept the security team on hand but restored voice discipline at the same time.

He also *adapted communication*. People tend to talk too fast and too loudly during a crisis. He spoke in a normal volume and soothing tone of voice. When people are loud our natural inclination is to match their tone and volume. Again, all behavior equalizes. Providers need to model the behavior we want to see. Crisis intervention expert Daniel Vega referred to this method as "reverse yelling". When people are being loud we need to get quieter, even at times getting very quiet so they can follow us down to a calmer state of mind.

The surgeon also *adapted his communication* by stating the obvious to his patient. People in altered states of consciousness and others who might have brain-based disorders such as autism or Alzheimer's syndrome, may struggle with understanding their circumstances. By telling his patient that he was in a hospital and that he had ingested pills and alcohol, helped fill in the blanks. He also spoke in short, direct sentences. He used his name frequently so he understood clearly that he was addressing him and not someone else.

Meeting urgent unmet needs is another technique that can normalize people in crisis. I've seen all sorts of behaviors stabilize after meeting just basic human needs such as toileting, hunger, or thirst. I've seen biting and spitting behaviors disappear after just giving a non-verbal patient a cup of water.

These five tactics: *reduce stimulation, separate and support, adapt communication, model calm behavior* and *meet urgent unmet needs* are tactics that complete the skill set Vistelar calls *Crisis Interventions*. In an age when brain-based disorders are growing in unprecedented numbers, providers will need to become more proficient in such a skill set, which requires a commitment to training and education for providers.

Human conflict is always a concern in the practice of healthcare, not only when serving patients who have brain-based disorders or psychiatric conditions, but for all patients experiencing a medical emergency or chronic medical condition. Limits on time and even space in medical facilities often ensure that conflict will occur, especially if policies are too rigid and providers too inflexible. Often we have to think outside the box to better serve patients and prevent conflict.

A woman with a severe headache presented at an emergency department, seeking help to manage her pain. None of her routine medications or anything she had tried was helping. As luck would have it, her headache flared up on a Friday afternoon. Now, over 24 hours later on a Saturday night, help from her family doctor was unavailable. Having suffered from severe and debilitating headaches for years, on rare occasions she had no choice but to seek help at an emergency room. This was another one of those nights.

Sometimes her headaches could last for days and the pain could be unbearable. Her headaches were more than a condition — they were an affliction; an affliction that had ruined her career, impoverished her life, and threatened her future. Over the years they had strained and even severed many of her relationships with family and friends.

Ultimately, they were at the root of a profound depression that had left her feeling hopeless and wrestling with thoughts of suicide. Still, that Saturday night she had enough hope left for one thing. She hoped for enough relief from her pain to eat without vomiting and sleep for a few undisturbed hours.

She had been through the E.R. process enough times to know what to expect. Depending on whom she got as a triage nurse, she would be treated with dignity and shown respect or treated like a drug addict. And depending solely on luck again, she hoped to draw a physician who would treat her with compassion and not suspicion. She'd been around the block enough to know that drug seekers are an issue at emergency rooms and that one of the symptoms they presented with was headaches. That is why she rarely sought help there. But this was just one of those nights when she just had to take that chance.

The waiting room was busy — crammed with patients, families and children. The television was blaring and the line was long. The bright florescent lights caused her to shield her eyes with her hands. Weak from the pain and an inability to eat, she could barely stand causing her to lean against the counter as she waited her turn at triage. It was all too familiar. She was in an environment that she would avoid under most circumstances, brightly lit, busy, and noisy. But she had to endure it if she was to take a chance at getting some help.

The triage nurse was obviously flustered, as she had been working diligently to cut down the line that kept pushing through the door. After checking in the woman asked, "Do you have somewhere I can wait that isn't so bright and noisy?"

"Sorry, you'll have to wait in the waiting room like everyone else," replied the nurse.

"How long do you think I will have to wait?" asked the woman.

"We have to take patients based on how sick they are, Ma'am, not on when they arrive," she replied, the implication being that her headache wasn't a medical priority.

"I understand that, but can you give me some idea on how long?" she asked.

"At least a couple hours," replied the nurse, tersely.

With that, she walked into the crowded waiting area. She tried to find an isolated corner, but there weren't any. She found a seat and sat with her head in her hands, covering her eyes. The blaring of the television and the laughter of children cut through her brain like an ice pick. She wished she had asked for a basin in case she needed to vomit as she felt waves of nausea washing through her stomach. Just then there was a commotion in the triage line.

"I'm not waiting in the f***ing waiting room! I'm sick!"

"I understand that sir, but we are very busy," replied the nurse.

"This is f***ing ridiculous!" he said. "I want to see a doctor right now!"

After a few more exchanges, she noticed a nurse rush forward from the back and escort the angry man back to an exam room. What she had witnessed was a familiar pattern in Emergency Department waiting rooms. Cause a scene or threaten the staff, and you won't have to wait like everyone else. The woman simply bowed her head and wept into her hands.

Healthcare workers are decent and compassionate people. The job they do is tough, both physically and emotionally. Stories like the one above are an exception in some facilities but routine in far too many others. When we train hospital staff to treat everyone with dignity by showing them respect, they not only learn to serve patients better, but they learn to care for themselves and each other better. And when we train to set the tone for how we deliver care, in a way that is caring and inclusive for all, we can prevent anti-social and violent behavior, instead of reinforcing and encouraging it.

Thank you for reading this book. I hope it gave you some tools that you can use to keep safe and be confident in conflict. The principles of violence recognition and response espoused herein cannot bear fruit without forward thinking and risk taking by healthcare providers and public safety professionals like Mike Thiel, the Director of Security at Children's Hospital of Wisconsin. None of them could have been developed or put into practice without the guidance of violence prevention and public safety experts like Bob Willis, Gary Klugiewicz, and Dave Young from Vistelar. The programs they instituted and the training they developed have had dramatic and lasting effects on the levels of violence experienced by the providers whose professional lives they have intersected. I join Mike, Bob, Gary and Dave in wishing every healthcare professional who reads this book, a long, happy and safe career.

Joel Lashley

Epilogue

by Mike Thiel

Whenever I enter a conflict situation that is playing out in front of a crowd, I listen for the onlooker who seems to be talking louder than the rest, whether it's yelling or simply talking to another person in a volume that's intended for others to overhear. I take the time to notice who is listening to that person. Non-verbal cues will always indicate when a person is listening. Cocking one's head to the side is the classic tell, even more so in adults because, as people age, their hearing diminishes in one ear faster than the other. I know I have to engage the active participants, but I'm looking for the "active" bystanders—the people who are listening intently and watching carefully, poised to run if things go bad, but not turning away just yet.

Group dynamics evolve as I take control of the situation. I know I have to offer the person who has lost control the opportunity to regain that control. But I also have to stop fear from developing in the herd. I watch for restlessness in the herd, those "active" bystanders who might move when that loud voice turns into hysteria. If the herd starts a stampede, it'll take a ton more time and effort to restore peace. But, if the herd feels safe, they're more likely to assist in restoring peace, whether by active participation or by passive acceptance that there is nothing to fear. Active bystanders (listeners) help me achieve the desired effect of restoring peace when they switch their listening from that loudest voice to my voice.

So, now let's broaden our horizons and think about all of healthcare as one big herd, in which we are all members. Empowered with our confidence in conflict, we are uniquely positioned, each and every one of us, to help create a culture incompatible with violence. Remember that maintaining peace in our little pasture of this enormous herd helps the "herders" next door maintain peace in their pasture. Also, realize we are one very smart herd. We have technology that connects us and we have a massive thirst for information about what's going on in other parts of the herd. Information, analysis and conclusions flow through our herd at the speed of light.

We've got to recognize that the healthcare herd is currently restless, as evidenced by the most recent OSHA report on violence in healthcare and social services.[2] The tasks necessary to create a healthcare herd incompatible with violence seem overwhelming, some might argue impossible. "We can't change all of healthcare." Indeed no single person or even large group of people can.

I believe a single drop of water raises the oceans. I'm sure there are scientists that can gracefully explain surface tension and cohesion to illustrate why I can't measure the Pacific Ocean rising from placing a single drop of water in the Atlantic. But here's a simple rational for my understanding, I can eventually fill a cup of water by dripping single drops of water in it. The oceans are simply a bigger cup. So while I can't measure it, I know it has to be true. We may have the viewpoint that healthcare is like the oceans and a single interaction can't make a measurable difference. We may have a hard time measuring it, but each interaction makes a difference. Healthcare is data driven, we'll figure out how to measure the difference along the way. Or better yet, we'll know we made a difference when it starts to get easier to see.

A simple statement; nothing changes if nothing changes.

If we draw the conclusion that creating a healthcare environment incompatible with violence is overwhelming or perhaps impossible, then that conclusion implies doing nothing. But, nothing changes if nothing changes. And most importantly, doing nothing is not an option. We can't escape or ignore conflict in healthcare. Every act of violence in our communities involves healthcare in some way. The healthcare herd isn't separate from the herd that is all of us. Something is changing because we are already doing something, whether it's by our own volition or by other's. If we create the perspective that each and every interaction ultimately creates the environment we desire, and that environment is one that is incompatible with violence, then we proceed into each interaction with confidence, respect and trust.

It will never, ever become better if we simply do nothing and let's be honest, all of us are trying to do something. The concepts in this book are not intended to be the magic pill, such that one swallow cures the patient. Just like filling a cup with single drops of water, take one of these concepts and try it in one situation, in one conflict and see if it works. It won't be perfect the first time; these skills aren't natural. Afterwards, debrief (talk) with someone that watched you. Discuss and analyze what you did and what was the outcome. Did it work? If the answer is "no", try something different. If the answer is "a little," then determine what you did that caused the little bit of success and do more of that. If the answer is "yes," then try to do that again in another difficult conversation. Analyze the second instance in the same manner. And, so on, until you feel you have enough repetitions to teach someone else. Have them go through the same process, until they get enough repetitions to teach another. Slowly, but surely, the environment will start to change. Each interaction, a single drop.

About the Author

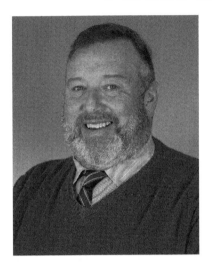

Joel Lashley has worked in public safety for over thirty years and, since 1991, has focused on healthcare security. Within healthcare, he has extensive firsthand experience in keeping the peace in hospitals, clinics and residential treatment facilities.

He currently works at Aurora Health Care where he supervises security operations for community clinics in Wisconsin. The largest employer in the State of Wisconsin, Aurora Health Care is an integrated healthcare provider with over 31,000 employees, 15 hospitals, over 150 clinic sites and more than 7.5 million annual patient encounters. Joel is also a Certified Consultant with Vistelar, a consulting and training institute that focuses on addressing the entire spectrum of human conflict at the point of impact — from before an interaction begins through to the consequences of how an interaction is managed.

Mr. Lashley is the author of many articles on topics ranging from providing care for people with brain-based disorders and psychiatric challenges, to managing patient prisoners in private healthcare facilities. He is in demand nationwide for his expertise in creating environments of care and clinical relationships that are incompatible with violence, resulting in better and safer working conditions for caregivers and higher customer satisfaction levels for patients.

As an award-winning educator and trainer, he has taught his principles for addressing healthcare violence (e.g., seven myths of healthcare violence, *Gateway Behaviors of Violence, Social Contracting*,

Crisis Interventions) to physicians, psychiatrists, nurses, healthcare security staff, social workers, law enforcement officers, corrections officers, residential care workers, and educators.

Mr. Lashley also provides training and consulting to healthcare professional organizations, hospitals and healthcare systems, crisis intervention training companies and law enforcement agencies, all of whom are concerned with the epidemic levels of violence in healthcare.

Can You Please Write A Review?

Thank you so much for reading my book! I really value your feedback so it would be wonderful if you could find the time to write a review on Amazon.

When you do this, please send me an email with the "By" name and date of your review so I can check out what you wrote and provide you with a free gift in return for your help.

Please send your email to: reviews@vistelar.com.

I'd Love To Hear Your Peace Story

Now that you've learned how to create an environment of care that is incompatible with violence, hopefully you've been able to use the skills you've learned.

If so, I'd love to hear your story.

To submit a story, please visit:

www.ConfidenceInConflict.com/peacestories

More Publications From Vistelar

Now that you have an understanding of what Confidence in Conflict means for healthcare professionals, please check out our other books in this series: **Confidence in Conflict For ...**

- Everyday Life
- Sports Officials
- Campus Life

Check out our many training manuals: **Conflict Management For ...**

- Everyday Life
- Campus Public Safety
- Law Enforcement
- Private and In-House Security
- Hospitals and Clinics
- Behavioral Health
- K-12 Schools
- Retail Loss Prevention & Security
- Public Utilities

All of these books and manuals are available on Amazon or can be purchased directly from Vistelar.

Members of Vistelar's team come from a wide range of professions and walks of life and, as a result, we have the ability to synthesize our conflict management methodologies with what happens in real life across many work and social environments. Therefore, please watch for other books and manuals in our *Confidence In Conflict* and *Conflict Management* series.

Joel Lashley

Learning Opportunities From Vistelar

Speaking

In-Person Training

Online Learning

Vistelar is a consulting and training institute focused on addressing the entire spectrum of human conflict at the point of impact — from before an interaction begins through to the consequences of how an interaction is managed. This includes non-escalation, de-escalation, crisis intervention and physical alternatives (e.g., personal protection, defensive tactics).

Vistelar clients include all organizations where human conflict has a high prevalence, such as law enforcement, health care, loss prevention, security, education, customer service and business. In addition the company provides training programs for everyday life (e.g., college students, sports officials, domestic violence).

Vistelar offers a wide range of training programs that address how to:

- Provide better customer service
- Predict, prevent and mitigate conflict
- Avert verbal and physical attacks
- De-escalate conflict
- Control crisis and aggression
- Handle physical violence

The results at the organizational level are:

- Higher levels of customer satisfaction
- Improved team performance, morale and safety
- Reduced complaints, liabilities and injuries
- Protected reputation, culture and business continuity
- Reduced harm from emotional and physical violence
- Decreased stress levels, lateral violence and bullying
- Less compassion fatigue, absenteeism and turnover
- Not having a damaging video show up on YouTube or the evening news

Vistelar's training is focused on the point of impact — the short period of time when disagreements, insults or gateway behaviors, such as swearing or aggressive posturing, can escalate to conflict and on to emotional and/or physical violence.

Vistelar trains "contact professionals" who directly interact with the general public or an organization's clients, as well as organizational teams and individuals who want to improve their performance and life quality by better managing conflict.

Vistelar's methodologies have been proven in real-world environments for over thirty years and are the subject of several books and training manuals in Vistelar's *Confidence In Conflict* and *Conflict Management* series.

Training is provided via speaking engagements, workshops, and instructor schools — using both live and online methods of instruction. Vistelar also hosts its *Beyond Conflict Conference* where attendees have the opportunity to learn the latest about how to effectively manage conflict.

Vistelar's vision is to make the world safer by teaching everyone how to treat each other with dignity by showing respect – via its continued efforts to be the world leader in point-of-impact conflict management training.

To learn more:

Call: 877-690-8230

Email: info@vistelar.com

Visit: www.vistelar.com

Get Immediate Access
To a Free Gift

As a thank you for purchasing and reading this book, Vistelar would like to provide you with a **free gift.**

Just go to the URL below to get immediate access.

www.ConfidenceInConflict.com/freegift

Here you can also:

- Access our Training Calendar with registration information for upcoming in-person training programs

- Access our listing of Online Training programs

- Learn about booking a Vistelar speaker at your next event

- Get information about contracting with Vistelar to provide a customized training program for your agency, company, organization or group

- Find out how to host a Vistelar training program at your facility and receive free slots in the hosted class

- Access our online shopping cart with Vistelar books, manuals, online courses, workbooks, apparel and other products

Joel Lashley

Made in the USA
Columbia, SC
22 February 2018